The Weight We Carry

The Weight We Carry

Navigating Life with Lymphoedema

KIERSTEN WALL

The Weight We Carry

ISBN: 978-1-78324-387-7

Dear Readers,

I am not a medical professional and I do not claim to be one. The purpose of this book is to reflect on my personal journey with lymphoedema. This includes the impact not just physically, but emotionally, mentally, and financially as well.

I hope to bring joy, hope, and inspiration to my readers.

Enjoy

CONTENTS

PROLOGUE

Everyone talks about the struggles of being a teenager, and sure, that's true. Still, nothing compares to the overwhelming experience of starting college: a new city, a new dorm, and an endless sea of new faces. But then once you enter the real world, you wish you could go back and be thankful for how easy it really was. Keeping a job, building a career, financial responsibility, maintaining a social life, keeping your sanity, finding love, as well as the stress caused by health and the nuisance caused by insurance companies. Some people may have it easier and some harder. We all have our own obstacles that we may or may not be able to handle. The weight of all this is overbearing.

My personal theory is that my obstacles began when I was sixteen. With the knowledge I have now, I believe I had stage one lymphoedema in my right ankle at this young age. Without a diagnosis and by following the wrong treatment approaches, I was doing everything I shouldn't do for this type of edema, so my limb worsened. But I didn't know anything about it until three years later when at stage two, it turned my life upside down.

Having lymphoedema isn't a walk through a park. It is more like a painful crawl through a heavily dense forest. Then, when you think you've gotten to a clearing, you get sprung up by a trap dangling from the limbs of the trees and forced into a stalemate to overcome yet another obstacle. Over the course of ten years, I gradually read the Old Testament. I enjoyed reading Exodus and how Moses led his people to the Promised Land. As I was reading about their journey and the obstacles they faced, I thought their journey of wandering through endless dunes of sand was an appropriate parallel to how I felt with my lymphoedema. Why was God punishing me? I was wandering for years to reach that "Promised Land," not exactly knowing what it looked like.

Some may read this, or even just look at it, and think, "Why her? Why her story? What is so special about her to write a memoir?" I'm not an actor nor a celebrity and nowhere near wealthy nor popular. I don't claim to be special, and I don't claim to be different, important, or the like. I do claim to be passionate, opinionated, honest, and ambitious. I am wealthy in knowledge, love, and friendship. I also think it is important to share my story, my journey, and experiences with others so they know they are not alone. This is not a weight loss journey; this is not a dieting journey. This is about facing daily obstacles and making the most of the life that God gave me, using what He gave me.

My mission is to make powerful statements of encouragement and positivity and to bring hope to those who are stuck in their well. The purpose of this book is to show how I am perfectly imperfect. I want to express the message to those around me that we are all perfectly imperfect. Whether you have lymphoedema or any other disease or illness, you are not alone. This is my story.

The First Symptoms

January 2014

I woke up for my 8:00am class. It was a normal start to the day. I have never been a morning person, but those were the days when I was severely not a morning person. You might have had better luck confronting a hungry alligator than crossing the path of my snapping attitude. Getting ready meant being half asleep and angry at the world. As I started getting dressed, I grabbed my jeggings; left leg in, great. Right leg going in, and…stuck? I looked down to find my knee grossly swollen. My calf and foot were twice the size they were the day before. There was no more shape to my knee and my ankle bone was nowhere to be seen. I called in my roommate who was a major in sports medicine and therapy. I do believe her words were, "Houston, we have a problem." Little did I know that day my life would change forever. Little did I know, overnight, I had stage two lymphoedema in my right leg, but we wouldn't know that diagnosis until six months later. Just like that, what were supposed to be the best years of my life instantly became the worst. My life had turned upside down.

As a student-athlete on my school's Division III softball team, I had access to the physical therapy room. I remember going to the athletic trainers the next day to show them my swollen leg. The pain was unusual to describe. At the time I wouldn't have said I was in agony, but my limb was certainly in discomfort: tight skin, redness, decreased mobility, heaviness, and pitting edema. It was an uncomfortable, confusing feeling having pressure against everything inside my leg. Naturally, from an athletic trainer's point of view, the first reaction was to ice it. So, for the next five months, I did. I iced and iced and iced to no avail. In fact, my leg was only getting worse (I know. Anyone with lymphoedema is probably screaming at me by now). After my softball practices and games, there would be a muffin top of skin draping over my knee where my pants and socks came together. Later, I would learn this was leaking lymphatic fluid building up due to the constriction of my apparel. My clothes were quite literally causing a beaver dam in my own body. It was gross, embarrassing, and I didn't know what to think of it.

I had a hard time in school, always did growing up, and college was no walk in the park either. In fact, it was more like a very long walk through hell. Unknowingly battling sleep apnea (diagnosed in 2016), ADHD, fainting due to vasovagal triggers, anxiety, and now a mysterious, chronically swollen leg, I was not okay. My leg didn't hurt in the way of being broken or sprained. It wasn't bruised and there were no signs of a blood clot, so I decided to wait until I was home for summer break to see my primary care physician. Already having failed three courses, I couldn't afford to miss any school and risk falling further behind.

Ironically enough, I did (and still do) happen to have swollen lymph nodes in my left groin. I discovered these at the end of the year in 2013, only a month before my right leg swelled up. Coincidence, some may say, but the doctors had no idea. Scientifically, there was no research to say whether the swollen lymph nodes and lymphoedema were correlated. Obviously, this is a concern when one finds lumps anywhere in their body. I had a fine needle aspiration of the nodes done, and it came back with no findings of anything wrong. They were swollen for no reason and I was told not to worry. I was advised to monitor them and bring it up if they got any larger. Despite this assurance, I was still confused because I thought lymph nodes only swelled when something was wrong? Don't lymph nodes swell when they are battling an internal war? Well, I'm not the one with the credentials, so I moved past these concerns fairly quickly.

The process of what came next was scary, confusing, discouraging, and exhausting. I do know how lucky I am to have been diagnosed in the time period I was as opposed to other patients. It normally takes years, or even a lifetime, for some to be diagnosed. It took me only a few months. I was (and still am) 4'11"and around 110 pounds. Visibly, my right leg was abnormally large and swollen; however, I was also not overweight in any capacity. I did not have any traumatic experiences to any internal nor external systems, and I had never undergone any kind of operation. This left every single doctor I saw at a loss of words. Each one running their special tests then sending me on to the next specialist. It was hard to say, "nothing is wrong with you," because thankfully there was visibly something wrong with me. My primary care physician and family nurse practitioner stood with me every step of the way. They became my home base in this great mystery we were trying to solve. They listened to me, believed me, and helped me to the best of their ability. I think I can safely say they were on the list with many others who breathed a sigh of relief when I finally got a diagnosis.

Starting with my primary care physician, Doctor M., I was referred for an x-ray, then shuffled to the gynecologist, reluctantly sent to a cardiologist, and dragged to a vein specialist. Each time, I returned to "home base," Doctor M. and Family Nurse Practitioner JK between specialist visits. My parents and I didn't take no for an answer, no matter how many appointments, phone calls, and consultations it took. I had multiple ultrasounds, palpation tests, and MRIs. This was all discouraging, but my last stop was at Vein Solutions in Stony Point to see a vascular surgeon. This is where everything changed.

I'll never forget when my mom and I were being taken back by the nurse. An older, petite lady looked at my mom and asked, "Do you have shorts to change into?" Meanwhile I am in shorts, not only because we were in the middle of our humid Virginia summer, but also because I knew my leg would need to be looked at. My mother looked at her and said, "Oh, I'm not the patient. My daughter is." This petite older lady looked at me and, with a look of genuine concern, said, "Oh, you poor thing. You're too young!" At this point in this miserable and depressing process I thought if I heard "Oh, you poor thing" one more time I was going to explode. I knew they all meant well by it and wished for me to be better, but as a nineteen-year-old who visibly had something wrong with her, that not a single specialist could figure out, sympathy wasn't exactly what I wanted to hear nor was it helping. I can't say I know for sure what I would have wanted to hear. I didn't want to be there at all. I didn't want anything wrong with me, and I certainly didn't want anything uncurable. Well, with this visit my one wish did come true. Finally, I got a diagnosis, identified by a vascular surgeon, and I will forever be grateful to him for knowing what lymphoedema is and how to diagnose it. However, that was all he could do. He wrote me a referral for an occupational therapist in town and said, "This is who you will see for management. You will have this for the rest of your life, and it will only get worse because there is no cure." As the weight of the unknown was lifted from my shoulders, I was not prepared for the emotional weight to come.

I left hoping it was all a nightmare and I would wake up back in January, at school perfectly normal again. I hoped he was wrong and wanted to get other opinions. I hoped for a lot of things but hoping wasn't getting me anywhere.

When I was diagnosed, I was told it was lifelong and incurable. The mindset given to us, right off the bat, was doom and despair. Why does it have to be this way? Why can't we be told the truth, but also be told it's manageable? How do we change the narrative from lifelong, incurable, and "it will only get worse" to feasible, treatable, and livable?

I really wish I could remember all the medical appointments I had the summer of 2014. I can find every planner for every other year in the last ten *except* that one. Did I throw it away because it was a reminder of the year from hell? Or it's very plausible it is hidden somewhere forever in the deep, dark depths of a corner in a box. I don't know and I will likely never find out.

My first appointment with my occupational therapist, let's call her CLT Bell, was interesting to say the least. I almost felt like I should have been at school instead of a medical appointment. I got a "Dos and Don'ts" sheet that was exactly what it sounded like, all the "Dos" and "Don'ts" of lymphoedema. There were examples on avoiding injuries to the skin. Don't walk barefoot. Avoid scratches from pets, other animals, activities, and the outside world. Avoid mosquito infected areas. It even specified the need to be careful when trimming toenails, to use an electric razor to shave affected areas, and to wear supportive shoes to avoid ankle injuries. Yet, how was I to do that when shoes aren't made wide enough for my swollen foot to fit in without it being 4 sizes too big? Avoid anything with fine needles. Avoiding heat was another "don't." So that means no more sauna, hot tubs, and laying out in the sun. That's not a fun one when you're only twenty years old. By then I was thinking, "I don't like this list." The "don't" list continues on to list things that can negatively impact the limb(s) including clothing, jewellery, and travel. As if I wasn't already discouraged enough, with every line I read all I got out of it was the feeling that my life was ruined.

In addition, I received a handout of an exercise program to do while bandaged. The purpose of this was to use the muscles to encourage the lymphatic fluid to pump. I was taught all about the bandages, their purposes, and how to wrap my legs. I even received pictures showing the steps! Another handout had instructions with pictures demonstrating how to perform self-manual lymphatic drainage (self-MLD) as well as how to perform deep abdominal breathing. As I said, I felt like I should've been in a lecture rather than an appointment at the "wound care center." My mom and I spent hours in these appointments with CLT Bell. Together we went three times a week for several weeks. The purpose was to educate me on the management tools to properly care for the swelling. I was also undergoing complete decongestive therapy (CDT). CLT Bell's primary objective was to drain my leg of fluid as much as we possibly could before measuring me for my very first set of compression garments.

Despite this grueling new routine I was forced to undergo, we had some pretty good laughs in our appointments as well as at home. You should have seen Mom and I trying to wrap my leg in the beginning. It's almost like learning how to tie your shoes again—start here, tail towards the pinky toe, cross over, figure-eight around the ankle, fifty percent overlap, next layer starts the opposite way, wrap around heel, you want it taut, but not tight, and so on. Figuring out the right pressure was something I struggled with for years. I wrapped either way too loose or *way* too tight. I had a very difficult time finding that happy medium.

When I left at the end of the summer to go back to school, everything was different. Friends had questions and wanted to make sure I was okay, but it was difficult explaining something I didn't even understand. My diagnosis journey wasn't over yet because I was in denial. Being a Division III athlete on the softball team, my life got even more difficult because I needed to wear compression garments all the time. If I had more knowledge, understanding, and acceptance of this diagnosis I think I would have been able to make it. However, that was not the case and I could not take care of myself. I found it in my best interest to end my softball career early. Do I wish I played all four years in college? Absolutely. However, at the time, I was failing a few of my classes, I was failing taking care of myself, and I didn't want to fail in my sport. I wanted the end to be my decision, not the lymphoedema's decision, and I wanted to end it on a good note.

Since I didn't understand my new disease, trying to explain it was always a long spiel. I was taking an equine anatomy class which took place once a week at the end of the day. One particular evening I decided to go to class wrapped in my bandages so I could go straight to bed afterwards. I was still self-conscious of all this compression stuff, but this was a very small class with those in the equestrian department who were already familiar with what I was going through. Plus, swelling is nothing new to horse people. Upon arrival, the vet noticed I had my leg wrapped and asked if I was okay. Getting prepared for my long spiel I started with, "I was just diagnosed with lymphoedema." Before I could go on any further, she interrupted, "Oh goodness, here prop your leg up! Do you need anything?" Saying I was shocked was an understatement. Not only did she know what lymphoedema was, but she knew what to do for it as well.

Ever since this encounter in 2014, every single equine veterinarian I have come across (which have been a lot) know all about lymphoedema. The further I studied horses the more I understood why. Horses have **thousands** of lymph nodes in their body as opposed to the six-hundred humans have. Lymphatic issues are a daily concern with horses. From manageable swelling standing in the stall, to the more severe cases of lymphangitis and cellulitis, it can even progress to equines developing lymphoedema. It is interesting that in my experience, large animal veterinarians appear to demonstrate a deep understanding of lymphoedema.

Five Stages of Grief

Denial: "an assertion that something said, believed, alleged, etc., is false" (Dictionary.com). As much as it was nice to have a name to my mysterious condition, it was super discouraging hearing that it was incurable and would get worse over time. I refused to believe it to be true. So, after all the appointments we went through to get an answer, we continued to seek second opinions. Unfortunately, this route got us absolutely nowhere. Shocker. Everywhere I went, the doctor would say, "I don't know what lymphoedema is, so I can't help you. I am sorry." How is it that no one knows about the lymphatic system? Clearly the lymphatics can have problems too, so why are there no specialists?

I went as far as having genetic testing. I did a research project in my equine breeding class in college. I wanted to learn more about how DNA worked and the possibilities of genetic mutations. So, the following summer, needing a break from disappointment, I did genetic testing at Virginia Commonwealth University (VCU) hospital. There, I was in a room with several different specialists, accompanied by med students, all at once. Was it intimidating? Yes. Did they ask a lot of questions? Yes. Did I know the answers to these questions?

No. None of them had seen this kind of pitting edema before and not one had heard of lymphoedema. Among the specialists present were a psychologist, an interventional radiologist, an orthopedic surgeon, a pediatric surgeon, and a plastic surgeon.

The final report of my genetic findings concluded, "Your lymphoedema appears to be primary and you do not have other clinical findings that are suggestive of a particular syndrome.... Thus, we have not been able to identify a genetic cause for your lymphoedema." The pathogenic variants known at the time that cause lymphoedema included "Milroy Disease, Hennekam Syndrome, Lymphedema-distichiasis Syndrome, Emberger Syndrome, autosomal dominant Lymphedema type 1C, microcephaly and chorioretinal dysplasia, and Lymphedema with hypotrichosis and telangiectasia" according to the final papers.

All in all, I saw one vascular surgeon, one vascular specialist, the slew of specialists at the genetic testing center at VCU, a board-certified phlebologist, several more ultrasounds and one final CT scan before I gave up on second opinions. As a result, I didn't want to face the diagnosis. I wanted to ignore it.

Anger: "a strong feeling of displeasure and belligerence aroused by a wrong; wrath" (Dictionary.com). I was angry. I was asking myself over and over again, "Why me, God, why me?" Anger was extremely difficult to overcome. I was angry at the world. I was angry with my body, and I was angry with everything I could no longer do. Nothing I did would ever be the same. I wasn't angry at people or family or friends. They didn't do anything wrong and the ones that were true stayed with me every step of the way. However, looking back, my demeanor towards the world was unfortunately taken out on everyone surrounding me. Everyone was patient and kind.

Through this tough time, I didn't lose a single friend nor family member. If any of you are reading this, I thank each and every one of you for sticking through it. I have some very special people in my life, and I know that. I knew that back then, but emotionally, I was going through too much to realize what I was doing and how I was acting.

Bargaining: "something, as a concession or inducement, that can be used in negotiating" (Dictionary.com). I wasn't one to go to church. I remember my family did occasionally attend church when my siblings and I were little. However, as we grew older, we got into sports and other activities which engulfed the weekends. But I wouldn't say we weren't, or aren't, godly people. Once we all moved out of the house my parents found the time to attend church on a regular basis. My excuses became the same as an adult. I am always busy on the weekends, and if I'm not busy, I really don't want to go anywhere. I don't get to do that often. Anyway, during this difficult time, I found myself bargaining with God. "God, I promise I will go to church every single Sunday for the rest of my life if I wake up free of lymphoedema." "God, I promise I will do anything you ask of me. Please rid me of this entrapment."

"God, I promise..."

"God, I promise..."

"God, I promise..."

Day after day, I wished I would wake up hoping it was all just a bad dream. I wished I would wake up and all this chronic swelling stuff was just my imagination. Obviously, this was never the case no matter how hard I pleaded. I wanted to bargain for my freedom again. It truly makes you see things from a different perspective. It truly makes you think about not taking advantage of the little things.

Enter depression. Depression: "the state of being depressed" (Dictionary.com). Why bother? That became my attitude. Why bother going out? Why bother taking care of myself? Why bother doing anything?

Why bother…?

Why bother…?

Why bother…?

I couldn't have any fun. My leg was going to hurt, putting me in a more miserable state. At this time, I became my biggest critic and my own worst enemy.

College was extremely difficult for me. It is difficult for me to learn in a lecture type-setting. I do best hearing the information, seeing the information, then applying the information. If I couldn't be hands-on with the material, I was going to forget it in five minutes. Countless times I wanted to get in the driver's seat of my car, head north, back home without looking back. The only thing that stopped me was that vein popping out of dad's forehead when he gets really mad. Assuming my dad wouldn't be too happy about me dropping out of college, I stuck with my misery and pushed on. It took me an extra semester to complete my degree because of the struggles I had with classes in the beginning, but I did eventually walk across the stage in one piece with a very expensive piece of paper. Compression garment and all.

I was extremely lucky to have a small group that stayed with me, my depressing attitude, and my struggles every step of the way. Shoot, I even ended up marrying one of them and, to this day, they are all a few of my favourite people. The group who lived above me were all humble and kind. They dealt with my tears, sorrows, and meltdowns from my lymphoedema as well as my mood swings and other issues. No matter what, they were always willing to welcome me with open arms providing me a safe place I could seek solace. My two closer friends on campus during these hard times kept me sane, on task, and in school. Because of these friends, I didn't feel so alone. They made me feel like I mattered. They couldn't help with my lymphoedema, and they couldn't relate to what it's like having this disease, but they could offer a shoulder to cry on, a buddy to sit with while pumping, a study partner curled up on the couch in the library, and encouraged me to do the things I did know at the time to take care of myself. The mental weight of living with lymphoedema is often heavier than the physical swelling and my friends were my rock.

The Turn of a Tide

I truly did not think I would complete my degree. As if I didn't already have a rough start my first year, now going into year two, after failing three courses, I have an incurable, chronic disease. Over the course of the next three years, I can't count how many times I wanted to get in my car, drive far, far away, and never return. I wanted so badly to quit school because I just couldn't handle it. I was living in pain with a swollen limb, I wasn't sleeping due to sleep apnea, and no matter how hard I tried, it was very difficult to keep up with life. The independency of college shows you who your real friends are. On campus, I had only a handful of true friends. I couldn't survive college on my own, but I did survive with them by my side. I may not have graduated on time, but you know what, who cares? We all have our own pace and obstacles and we shouldn't feel pressured to complete an entire degree in any specific time. I remember the day of my graduation, after everyone had their moment walking across the stage the president of the university congratulated us all. I threw my arms in the air. Holding my new diploma, I turned around and spotted my mom giving my dad a hug. I think they also knew this was very difficult for me. They knew I tried *so* incredibly hard. I started out as

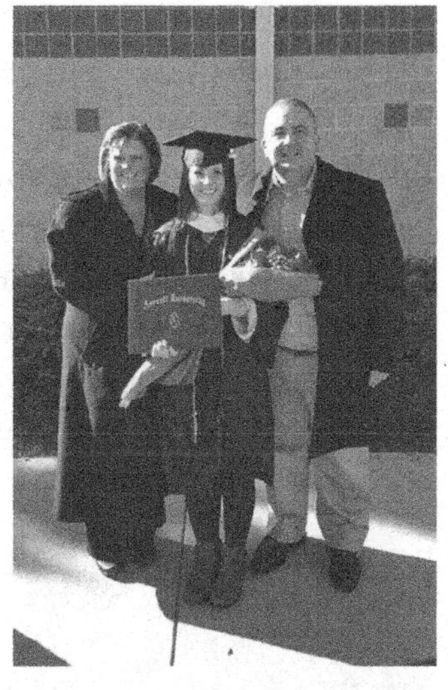

a C average student in high school—back when it was an eight-point grading scale—to a failing student my freshman year of college. With a little bit of help from my friends, my professors, and the university, I turned into an A/B student the second half of my college career. One of these friends who helped me survive turned out to be my future husband and he actually ignored me the most!

After my diagnosis, I started searching lymphoedema on Instagram. I followed other patients just like myself, as well as organizations that would put out information and awareness. As I followed more pages, I really enjoyed coming across the posts, but there was just one problem. The lymphoedema posts were getting lost amongst others I followed on my personal account. This led to the creation of my lymphoedema Instagram, *@8furlongs_of_lymph.* At the time I did not know this social media page would change my life. I still occasionally look back to my first post in 2018.

> *"The tide will* ***turn*** *as long as you're willing to go against the waves"*
>
> –KIERSTEN ESTES

When I posted it, the emotions were much deeper than just lymphoedema. At the time this picture was taken, a year and a half earlier, it was the most difficult time in my life for reasons I can't explain. I was nine hundred miles away from home and family, and I had no friends. The cherry on top of this emotional and depressing roller coaster was the lymphoedema making the physical and mental exhaustion worse. My right leg quickly worsened with each passing day. When I started wishing I'd get hurt just to escape the environment, my parents essentially flew down and told me I was going home, even if they had to kidnap me. My parents strongly encouraged me to put in a two-week notice.

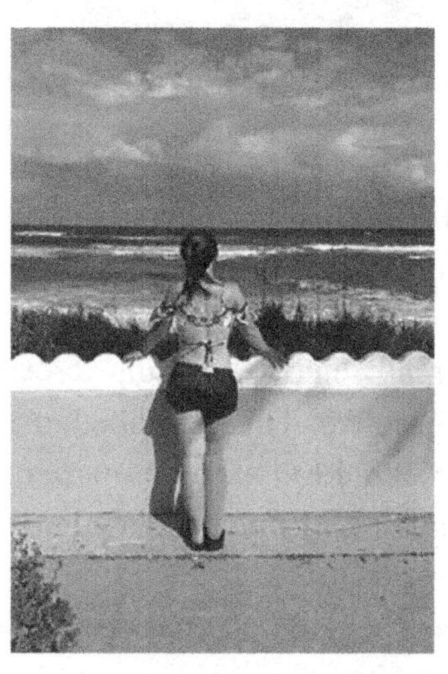

That is when this particular picture was taken, as I was looking out at the waves off the sandy shore. Looking out at the sea it was so calm and the water so flat beyond the waves. But on the shore, the waves were crashing on the sandbar one after the other, determined to keep anything from disrupting the calmness that lay beyond them. Looking out at the waves I realised I had to go against them for things to get better. I had to do something scary to get away from all the pain. I had to face it head on. Or else I would be stuck in the crashing surf allowing myself to get beat up. Two weeks and one day later, I was on my way home. I was physically incapable of driving at that point, so my mom booked a one-way flight down to drive me back home—with the unsafe vehicle I ended up having to buy on a whim after my beloved Jeep broke down for good.

I could also relate this quote to my lymphoedema. For so long, I was depressed and in a state of denial and not taking care of myself. I was stuck in the surf, allowing the disease to knock me down. I was drowning. However, I started to educate and take care of myself. My mindset shifted from, "why is this happening to me" to, "what can this teach me?" I went full force against the waves, and it made a difference! The sea on the other side was beautiful. I made it through and the tide turned for me. I went against the waves and everything became calm in my life. Everything became better.

You hear so many unfortunate and nasty things regarding social media, such as how people these days use and abuse it while hiding behind a computer screen in the comfort of their own home to make others' lives miserable. I am extremely fortunate I have yet to come across any negativity or nasty comments on my posts or sent to my direct messages. Not only have I not received any negativity, but over the years I have been overwhelmed with positivity, comfort, and understanding. This platform has given me incredible friendships all over the world.

Beyond the platform, there have been my friends, my family, my husband, and his family as well. There are my parents who would not take "no" for an answer at all the doctor appointments. They never hesitated to help by providing any compression or tools needed while I was on their health insurance. They also provided a safe home where I didn't need to feel guilty for the help I required nor embarrassed for the constant meltdowns I had. Even after moving out at the end of 2021, there have been many occasions I needed something from their house or they would run errands for me to help take a load off my shoulders. They knew how difficult some aspects of life could be for me, especially driving. After moving out, I lived an hour away from them, yet they were always offering to go out of their way to run an errand for me and meet me halfway to help me with my needs and limitations. Sometimes I dislike that they are such awesome parents, because when they offer to go out of their way it is hard to say no. My brother and his wife have been supportive and always willing to help find information if they can. They also have three beautiful girls who are growing up with my bandaging and compression being a completely normal thing. They don't ask, "Why? Why? Why?" They take the answer as it is and ask if they can help roll bandages or put my tools away. Then there's my husband, who even before marriage showed how much he loved me "through sickness and in health." Lymphoedema inadvertently affects him too. Because of my disease, he does all the cooking for us. Sometimes he has to do more errands or take care of things out of the way because I'm having a bad leg day and can't do it. He rolls my bandages on a daily basis and helps to keep it all put away and organised. In addition, he never complains about all the driving he does since I can't really contribute. My husband is always asking what I need help with and what he can do to make it easier on my legs. He was raised to be humble and kind. He is selfless and always puts my needs first. I wouldn't have the attitude nor emotional stability I have today without him. He helps get me through and makes life so enjoyable, lymphoedema or no lymphoedema.

My long-time friends from childhood into adulthood also stayed by my side throughout my whole journey. When I was going through grief and denial, you could say I dropped off the face of the earth. I didn't reach out to anyone. I was miserable and just didn't care to put forth the effort to try to stay in touch. Plus, having that extra weight to carry around was exhausting. There were times I could've gone out and had fun, but I really didn't want to put forth the effort to socialize. Most of my spare time was spent at home sitting around throwing myself a pity party.

As a kid, one is so innocent and worry free. That's such a great thing and sometimes I am jealous of the little ones who don't know the real world yet. But one day all kids grow up and learn the truths of the world around them when they are mature enough to understand. Unfortunately, there is no way to tell the future and know to take advantage of the little things. If I could go back in time, I would tell myself to enjoy the physical freedom and to appreciate the fresh air on the skin of my legs. Because one day I wouldn't have that anymore. I wish I could go back and soak up all those beach trips splashing in the sea, or slide into second base one more time without a care for scrapes and burns, or even sleep curled up in a ball with no compression pushing against the back of my knees. I would do anything to have these feelings one more time.

As I began to accept this fate and learn the tools to take care of myself, my occupational therapist, CLT Bell, talked to me about a pneumatic compression device. We scheduled a trial of this twelve-chamber compression pump through Tactile Medical. We did this in the summer of 2015, so I was about eighteen months into the disease and twelve months after receiving the diagnosis. At the completion of the one-hour session with my right leg in this device I saw space between my toes for the first time in eighteen months. *For the first time in eighteen months* the swelling had **visibly** gone down, I had space between my sausage-like toes and there was a visible shape to my leg again. The result was jaw-dropping. The before and after measurements were recorded for this successful trial and all paperwork was sent to insurance to obtain my own device, which cost thousands.

Three months later, I received a letter of denial from the insurance stating they did not see it as medically necessary. I had been warned to expect this, so with the help of Tactile Medical and CLT Bell, we quickly put in our appeal stating why it was medically necessary along with its impact based on the trial measurements. The extra work is a nuisance, but it was required to fight for my health. Then, we waited. Around Christmas-time, we received a letter in the mail. I was excited and nervous all at the same time to open it. My parents read it out loud: I had been denied again as it was still considered medically unnecessary. I was devastated. During the months waiting for this, my right leg had been worsening and getting more painful. As 2016 began, the denials continued and my emotional health declined. Finally, in April, nine months after the trial, insurance approved a trial three-month rental for the pneumatic compression device. This was the most inconvenient time possible. I was finishing my second to last semester in college, then heading straight to Kentucky for a life-changing internship. The three-month rental would end in another state, far from home, help, and my medical team. The challenge continued.

My internship was the absolute coolest experience I have ever had. It was at one of the top racing facilities in the world. I was in the training division under the trainer and assistant trainer at their private track on the property. Apart from observing training, I learned all about rehabilitation, medication, veterinary observation, and caring for thoroughbreds in race training. It was incredible. However, I was working an intense schedule of fourteen hours a day, six days a week. You really have to love it to be in the racing industry, and boy, was I loving every single minute of it, except for my leg. If you're thinking, "You have lymphoedema. How did you survive those hours?" The answer was pure heart and my twelve-chamber pump rental. My leg was full, heavy, and very much still there the entire summer. It was a burden. But I will say I fully believe I would not have survived that summer without my pump. Each day I woke up at four o'clock in the morning to be at the farm by four forty-five. I worked my thirteen to fourteen-hour day with a nap during my lunch break so I could prop my leg up for a while. Getting home, I was very thankful to have a roommate who had already finished her workday and made dinner. I did everything I could to help shop for groceries and keep the kitchen clean. I would take a shower, fall asleep in the pump, wake up to put a night garment on, then go back to sleep for the night before the sun went down. I'd wake up the following morning to do it all over again for eleven weeks. I can only imagine how much better it would have been without lymphoedema.

The Time In Between

2017-2023

The summer of 2017 came around and I was enjoying a calm, sunny day out on the boat with my husband. He likes to fish, so I would try to sit with him while he enjoyed his hobby when my right leg could tolerate it. It's very difficult for me to do the things he loves because we learned the hard way that I get gut-wrenching motion sickness. On this particular day, it was different. I was wearing my Rainbow flip-flops on the boat when suddenly the left flip-flop no longer fit. We were at the mouth of the Neuse River, where the river was several miles wide, and we were a good distance from the house. It looked like my fear of lymphoedema affecting other parts of my body may be coming true. My left foot was so swollen; I was in awe. I could feel the skin stretching and tightening as it grew in size.

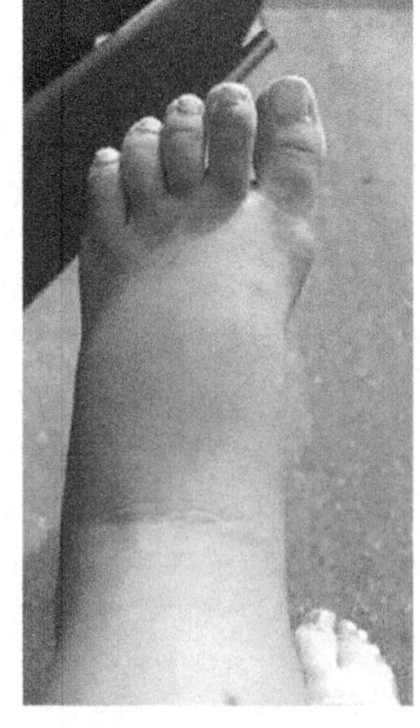

Here I was, finally past denial and accepting lymphoedema in my right leg, and now I wanted to deny this was happening in the left. Thankfully, by now, I had some knowledge. Knowledge is power and this superpower of mine came in handy. Despite desperately not wanting to, I had started wearing off-the-shelf circular knit garments to have on hand for my "bad" leg. Little did I know they would eventually be used for the "good" leg.

Pushing through the negative mindset all over again was not easy. Even though I had accepted lymphoedema by this time, this did knock me down several steps. Do you ever feel there's always something in life and you can't catch a break? You get past one problem or important matter, but as soon as you get a moment to sit down and breathe, another matter comes up and off you go again. That's how lymphoedema feels every single day. Each day brings a new struggle or battle with my own body. A different routine and a different way the swelling will respond to the therapy. Naturally I emailed CLT Bell absolutely freaking out. Bless her soul for being so patient with me over the years

Life with bilateral lymphoedema became so different. On a positive note, I've found it incredibly interesting to learn about the differentiating care requirements for each leg. My right leg (the "bad" leg) has always preferred a little extra tension against the limb and the biggest problem area is my calf. I find that all the extra foam pieces and tools under the wraps don't help very much. On the other hand, my left leg (the "good" leg) prefers a little less tension against the limb and the biggest problem areas are my foot and ankle. My foot loves all the extra foam and padding under the bandages. It is so unique having two completely different worlds within my own body. I always understood lymphoedema will appear different for everyone. As far as I can tell, it is one of the unknown mysteries of the disease. Some may respond better to night garments and others may not. Some may respond better to surgeries and some may not. Some may have the disease below the knee while others may have it in the whole limb. But what has been a learning curve for me has been the differences of the same disease in two different quadrants of my body. Despite the differences, I am grateful that both of my limbs have responded remarkably well to every surgery I've undergone. Each surgery was a lot to ask of my body. Using the tools I already had, I was able to sustain the left leg, likely stage one, for a little while. With my knowledge, I was able to keep it under control for two whole years with circular knit garments before I started my surgical journey and was diagnosed with stage two bilateral lymphoedema.

Does anyone talk about the stresses of life? Stressors may include working a full-time job, maybe multiple jobs, trying to eat healthy, exercising, home chores, having a social life, keeping yourself together, and finding time for family. When are we supposed to take care of ourselves? Or find the extra time needed to take care of a disease or illness? I finished reading *Lymphoedema United: You Are Not Alone* compiled by Amy Rivera and Matt Hazledine. I recognised several things about everyone's journeys. We all have our own paths, yet they still seem so similar in different ways. I could relate to everyone's beginning of lymphoedema. When we were diagnosed, we were told it is lifelong and incurable. The mindset given to us immediately is doom and despair. Earlier I asked, "Why does it have to be this way?" but what if it doesn't have to be? We can still be told the blunt truth, but also be told it's manageable. How do we change this narrative from lifelong, incurable, and "it will only get worse" to "feasible, manageable, and livable?" To answer this, we speak up. We use our voices. We let others know they can thrive. We let others know they can survive. We let others know it is possible to conquer the lymphoedema. We let others know they are not alone. Forming bonds and friendships with other patients all over the world has helped me get past the negative mindset and misery. Lymphoedema is a disease, not a choice. But it is my choice on how I react and behave due to the disease. It's up to me, and only me, to change the narrative for myself instead of dwelling on what I can't have or what I can't feel.

As I mentioned before, I thought my life was over. Due to the negative outlook I received at my diagnosis, I believed I would never find success or happiness in my lifetime. It wasn't until I pushed through the crashing waves, when I chose to change my mindset to "I am going to figure this out." I wanted to be in horse racing, but I didn't know how to get there. For my equine careers class in school, I interviewed an exercise rider and a pony rider. I wanted to be a jockey, but becoming one was far beyond my reach. When I had the chance to give it a try, it only took a few horses to see the lymphoedema was making it physically impossible to fulfil my dream to be a rider. So, I set out with the mindset, "How can I be in racing and have a positive impact for the horses, but still cater to my physical needs?" I was a history major and my only work experience was working as a horse groom. At this point in 2019, when I knew my career needed to change, I didn't know what I wanted to do, what I wanted to be, nor how to become it. So, just like the actor Johnny Depp, I became everything. Johnny Depp played a pirate, a wizard, King Louis XV, the Mad Hatter, an officer, and even a chocolatier! The list goes on for this A-list actor and he successfully crushes any type of role that he is in. Somehow, I tend to get myself thrown into things at full speed instead of gradually easing into them. I started riding horses as an adult while having no clue how to trot or handle young Thoroughbreds. But over a few short years I worked Thoroughbred auctions, handled Thoroughbreds on a farm, became a published photographer, and then a published author. My list isn't quite as long as Mr. Depp's, but I guess you could say I like a challenge. Every step I have taken in the last ten years has been vital for getting the job I now have today. I landed my forever dream job—promoting and advocating for Virginia Thoroughbred racing. I am on cloud nine and I, one hundred percent, have my lymphoedema to thank for it. I am involved with everything I have always wanted to do and I honestly wouldn't be here if it wasn't for this disease. If I had not developed lymphoedema, I more than likely would have gone off to be a jockey or an exercise rider. I am sure I would have loved it and been happy with that career path, but the work I have now is so fulfilling and gives my husband peace of mind that I don't have a career where there is an ambulance following closely behind.

During my bachelorette dinner in 2023, one of my bridesmaids had an insightful question, "What was the moment you knew he was the one?" At the time, I didn't have the truest answer to this on the fly. There had always been little signs over the years, so I responded with one of those little moments. However, it wasn't until after the fact when *the* moment hit me. The moment in my life that deserved all the glory as the answer to this question. I was a few months into my job as the payroll clerk at the racetrack. At the time I thought this was going to be it. I had reached my dream of working at a racetrack and I felt like I was part of the racing industry. (Obviously this changed over the next few years). I was on cloud nine. Warmer weather had finally arrived in Virginia. Trey was looking for a new job so that he could be closer to me. We had been in a long-distance relationship for four years. Everything felt like it was finally falling into place, and on this particular day I was just in a really happy mood. I was driving back home—to Mom and Dad's—with the windows down belting to Spotify through the car. Then it came on, the song "Here I Am" by Bryan Adams. Every horse girl reading this right now will probably know exactly what movie this is from—*Spirit: Stallion of the Cimarron.* In the movie, this song represents life. Young Spirit has just been born and he is saying hello to the world in "the place where I belong." When the song reached the chorus, "It's a new world, it's a new start" I completely lost it. There I was driving on I-64 bawling my eyes out as the song continued. In that moment, it had a whole new meaning for me. It no longer represented the new life of this colt who would grow up to be the stallion of his herd, but a meaning of a life worth living. A life worth living with this very special human being. "A new day, in a new land" was waiting for us as Trey mentally prepared himself to move away from his home state that he knew and loved, but he loved me more. By now, I had been through a few surgeries and my legs were doing better. It felt like a new start for me, and I felt so alive. That's when I knew he was the one.

Dealing with lymphoedema has accelerated my personal growth and maturity significantly. I had an extremely difficult time in college. I worked extremely hard to get good grades. I would show up, take notes, and study for hours and hours, but I needed to apply the information in order to retain it. Maybe that's why I found my niche in the horse industry. Despite knowing the information, I simply did not test well. Therefore, my main focus was school. Most young adults have at least one part-time job while attending university. I am fortunate that my parents were able to afford me a college education that allowed me to focus on my studies and my lymphoedema without the added stress of having to work. But truly, if I had been made to work as well as attend classes, I would have failed. When my leg blew up in my second year, I had too much on my plate to worry about. I had a disease I was not able to obtain information about, I was fighting insurance to get the necessary means to manage said disease, and, as a twenty-year-old, I was losing physical capabilities. It was a terrible time.

I am thankful my parents took care of my college education. Yes, it would have taught me a sense of financial responsibility and a taste of what it would be like as an adult with bills to pay and a job to manage. However, I had other challenges to face that most young people don't. I had to figure that out entirely on my own. I had a different weight on my shoulders hiding from within.

Anesthesia, Scalpel, Action

On July 29, 2018, something compelled me to create a second Instagram account for only lymphoedema posts and information. I needed a place to see all things lymphoedema without nonrelated posts getting in the mix. I needed to know if I really was alone in this world. This was hands down the best decision I have ever made and the best thing I could have done for myself. My Instagram has become my therapy, my advocacy, my connection to other Lymphies,—those who have been diagnosed with lymphoedema— and my opportunity to keep up with findings and information in the lymphoedema community. This is also how my surgical journey began.

Soon enough, I found other people with lymphoedema all over the world! I began following their accounts and scrolling through the posts. I began creating my own content and received comments and support from others who know exactly what I was going through. I had an overwhelmingly positive response while connecting with others all over the world. For the first time with this disease, I found others who could finish my own thoughts and sentences. It opened a whole new door to overcome the five stages of grief. It didn't take long before I started seeing posts about surgeries being performed, not necessarily to cure but significantly reduce the excess volume in affected limbs. I began doing my own research and became very interested in seeing if I could be a candidate. The only problem was how few surgeons in the world were doing these surgeries. The first one I discovered was located in Italy; this was financially out of the question. Continuing my research, I found a couple in the United States: one in California and one in Ohio. By now, I had started becoming more open to my parents about my lymphoedema, how it made me feel, and how all the interactions on Instagram excited me. They have given me every ounce of support since the very beginning and always wanted to help. As much as they wanted me to get better, California and Ohio were still too far for what we could afford and accommodate. If you know anything about me, you will learn quickly that I don't back down. I get this lovely trait from my father. And, thankfully, he didn't back down either. He wanted nothing more than his baby girl to not be in pain, so he began his own research. You see, a father has this internal responsibility to protect and provide for his family. My father made sure we had a roof over our head, clothes on our backs, and food in our bellies. However, he couldn't protect me from my lymphatic system. He couldn't protect me from my legs growing larger.

Through casual conversations, my mom got a lead from one of my sister-in-law's relatives who knew about someone being treated in Pennsylvania. My dad researched from there and, lo and behold, there was a plastic and reconstructive surgeon doing this specialised work for lymphoedema only 350 miles away in Baltimore, Maryland. This was more than doable. This was the start of something new and all because my parents talked to others about my lymphoedema.

I remember having to send a letter to the hospital to see if I would even qualify to see them for lymphatic testing.

Then, based on the testing, I would have a consultation with a surgeon. With multiple doctor visits on record, several years of occupational therapy, and having genetic testing done, it wasn't too difficult to get my first appointment for a lymphoscintigraphy. This was my first, of what would become many, experience of having dye injected between my toes. I remember this moment all too well. They numb the skin of course, but that's not where it hurts. There is excruciating pain internally while the dye is being injected. Thankfully, it doesn't last long, maybe thirty to sixty seconds after the injection, but still in the moment it was agonizing. With this being my first experience, I had absolutely no clue what to expect and I already despise needles. Before we began, I was asked if I was ready. I thought this was a strange question. I didn't come all this way to not be ready. As soon as the nurse started injecting, I screamed. I quickly stopped screaming, not wanting to disturb the other patients on the other side of the walls or the people in the waiting room down the hall, including my mother. The nurses hesitated, looked at me almost in a frightening way, and asked, "Are you okay?" I then yelled, "No, I'm not okay, don't stop!" The injections had to be done between every toe so at that moment I wanted it done as quickly as possible. Turns out the hesitation was concern because they were used to patients screaming in pain (spoiler alert, that time did eventually come for me during future tests). They even went so far as to find my mother to tell her that I had taken the injections better than anyone else. To which, knowing me, my mother did not believe them, in a loving way of course. She replied, "**MY** daughter? Are you sure you're talking about the right patient?" I walked away from this finding it truly hysterical.

Anyway, the lymphoscintigraphy test showed and confirmed a disruption in my lymphatic vessels only in my right leg. The final conclusion also noted an abnormal lymphatic distribution through the left lower extremity. The results gave me the green flag to schedule a consultation with the surgeon. I truly never thought I would be so excited for not only surgery, but surgical interventions that were past the experimental stage, but still not widely known in the medical field.

January 2019
Baltimore, MD

I couldn't have been more enthusiastic to be going to a doctor's appointment. This wasn't just any appointment; it was one for my lymphoedema and with the very first licensed physician (MD) I could see specifically for the swelling. I'll never forget my very first interaction with the doctor who specializes in reconstructive procedures. The nurse walked me back, took my vitals, and set me up in a room. Being in the plastic surgery office of the hospital, I noticed breast silicone pieces on the counter. As a woman I didn't think anything of it. After a minute, a very well-dressed man knocked and came in. He glanced my way and casually said, "I'll just get these out of the way. We will be with you in just a moment." And he scooped up the silicone pieces and awkwardly walked out. I don't know why I found this so funny, but I did. Moments later, the same very well-dressed man (the surgeon), his physician's assistant, and a nurse entered the room. They introduced themselves and prepared to inject dye between my toes. This was to look at my lymphatic system on a closer scale with an ICG lymphography test. This was the best test to finally get answers and see the flow for myself. The injections between the toes were excruciating. Injection one, deep breath, and here we go again.

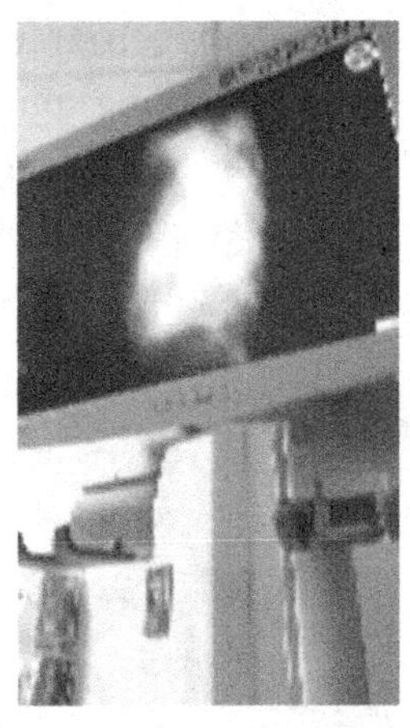

This time there was screaming, and my body couldn't handle it. I faintly got out, "I am going to pass out." With a history of this I knew it was coming. The bed had to be laid down.

For the first time in five years, I finally had an answer. With a confirmed diagnosis of stage two lymphoedema, we discussed my surgical options. By now I had researched all three surgeries in my own time. The lymphovenous anastomosis (LVA), suction assisted liposuction (SAL), and the lymph node transfer (LNT). We talked about each one and I expressed my concerns about the LNT. He professionally addressed my concerns while also respecting my hesitations about the procedure. He assured me that we would not discuss this route, at least not for now. He didn't say it to me in a "you're wrong" kind of way, but in an educational and a "it's not the right path right now" kind of way. Regardless, this wasn't the route he wanted to take until all other avenues had been exhausted. After this visit, I had surgery scheduled for the LVA in my right leg to take place in only three months.

April 2019
Baltimore, MD

I rode with my husband to Baltimore for my very first surgery. We drove separately from my parents because he could only stay for the one day, whereas my parents and I stayed two nights. We kept up with one another the entire drive up from

Richmond, getting to the city at dinner time. This was on a Sunday. Parking split us up, and my mom and dad got into the restaurant first. I had until midnight before I was cut off from eating. We ate at the Cheesecake Factory at the Inner Harbor. Always a good choice! I remember having a splendid evening and being way too excited to sleep. You know you are desperate for a resolution when you are excited to be cut open.

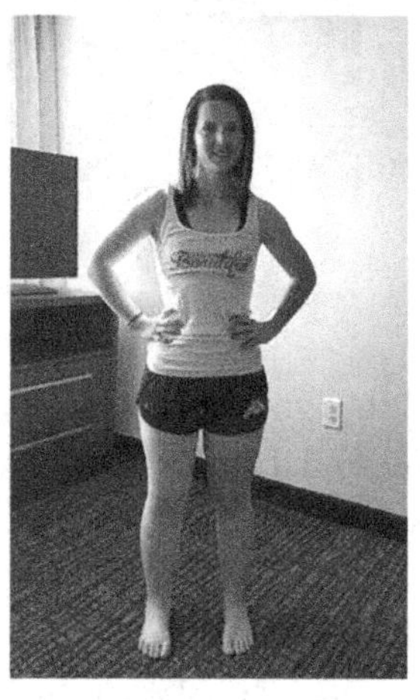

The morning went as normal. I got ready, took before photos, and was anxious to go when I got a phone call. The hospital called to say the appointment before mine was cancelled and I was welcome to get there sooner. I told them we were on the way! We stayed at the Renaissance, just a few blocks down, so we started walking. It was a comfortable spring morning for a quick walk to the hospital.

I woke up mid-afternoon with the intense feeling of fresh wounds all snuggled up in dressings. The successful operation took about four hours. Dr. Aliu was hoping for multiple connections, but he was only able to achieve one strong connection. One is better than none, and he was extremely optimistic. This was in my right leg and I honestly felt great. It hurt, but I wasn't in any unbearable pain. If anything, I was having more pain and issues with my throat than the leg that had just undergone surgery. I had no nausea from the anesthesia and my stomach felt great, so I was cleared to eat. I was starving, so I had asked for a chicken wrap. My father happily went out in the city traffic to get us Red Robin for dinner per my request. I took my first bite, but I quite literally couldn't chew nor swallow. Apparently dry throat is a common side effect. My throat was so dry because I had no saliva to break down the food. I was awfully sad and felt bad sending my dad to get food that I was not able to eat. Attempt number two—a smoothie and milkshake were brought back. I drank both, and, in that moment, it was the best meal I ever had. Having surgery is some hungry work!

As an outpatient operation, it was only a few hours before I was being discharged and sent home. Trey parted ways, going back home with the peace of mind I was okay. Mom, Dad, and I went back to the hotel for the night before putting me in the car for the four-hour drive back to Richmond. That night I was very comfortable after being graciously accommodated by the hotel with lots of pillows and a second milkshake from Dad before going to bed.

Did I mention I was feeling good and not in a whole lot of pain? Well, that drastically changed at four o'clock the following morning. All the hospital drugs I was given the day before had worn off and I was feeling all of the pain. We were very much unprepared for this as it was not until that moment that we realised we had no Tylenol—the only painkiller I was allowed to take. Dad insisted on going to the 7-Eleven across the street. With the crime rates in the area, I was worried about him walking outside while it was still dark and pleaded with him not to go. Now, is a father who is seeing his baby girl in pain going to listen? No. He marched his way over and came back safe and sound with the goods. We got some medicine in me and I dozed back to sleep.

I rested at home for only a few days before I was able to go back to work. Luckily, I was only working part-time and my employer was very understanding of my fragile state, including the fact that I was walking around with crutches for support. Life went on, and I noticed very positive improvements to my physical well-being. Now, we just needed to get all that excess fluid out of my leg.

The third day after my surgery was an experience like no other. At first, I was really embarrassed by this matter, but now I am more open. The constipation was probably by far more painful than the surgery itself. Everything was there, but it was more than my body could handle. My intestines were ready to get rid of the waste; however, it was too difficult. I was not warned that anesthesia does this, so I was not prepared. I had not been taking any preventatives to help, so I was in agony. My dad stayed home from work, but he couldn't really do much. After a much-needed recommendation, he went to the store for magnesium. This made the matter worse. (I will spare you the details). It may have taken hours, but the relief finally came. This was a valuable lesson for me. In future cases I knew to start preparing days in advance to help lessen the effects of constipation. The lesson here is when going under ask your doctor about constipation, drinking lots of water, and eating fiber-rich foods. It may help!

That summer, I had the experience of a lifetime. I began working in racing operations at the revitalised horse track in my state. I worked seventy to eighty hours per week during the racing season. This is when I realised how much the surgery truly benefitted my life. My right leg was less heavy and more capable of the long work hours. I was amazed at how manageable the swelling became. For the very first time in four years, I started to think, "I can do this."

March 2020
Baltimore, MD

My parents and I packed up the car and headed to Baltimore once again for surgery number two. I'll never forget the moment leaving the driveway. Honestly, it's quite sad. At the time, I was 25—only two months away from turning 26. Driving up our street my father said, "You turn 26 soon and won't be able to stay on my insurance." He said this in a very sad and serious manner. I chuckled, responding, "Dad, normally parents are excited to have their grown children off their benefits." From the driver's seat he looked at me in the rear-view mirror and dead serious said, "I would be if you were healthy." It really saddened me that my parents not only had to worry about my health, but also bear the financial strain of insurance—especially with a life-altering disease that insurance refuses to support. It was a concern we shouldn't have had, but nonetheless, onward we went.

Back in Baltimore, we met my husband there (year two of surgeries). This surgery was more involved because the lymphoedema had now developed to stage 2 in my left leg. This time, our plan was to perform the SAL procedure on my right leg and the LVA procedure on my left leg. This time it would take twice as long as the previous surgery, approximately eight hours.

The surgery was once again a success. By now, I had gained experience keeping myself comfortable immediately after waking up from anesthesia. Scarred by the sore throat from the year before, I made my first request for a milkshake as soon as possible. The order was sent to the hospital kitchen. We came with Tylenol and I knew to stay hydrated while also eating fiber-rich foods. The only area I had failed in my preparations for this surgery was the lack of expectation on how much more painful this surgery would be. Lord have mercy, the pain was unbearable compared to anything I had experienced in my life.

I got wheeled across the whole hospital to my room. This was so much fun! Who can resist a little moment in the spotlight every now and then? The room they had available for me overnight happened to be on the cardiology floor with patients recovering from heart surgery. When I arrived, there was a lot going on. All chaos ensued. My family came walking in right behind me, but stayed out of the way. A young man was there to help move me from the operating room bed to the new bed as well as the nurse on shift. I was loopy waking up from anesthesia and the nurse was frantically speaking to me. "What went wrong? Why are you on the cardiology floor?" and "Patients with your surgery don't stay overnight." I was instantly irritated. She must not have had experience seeing many lymphoedema surgeries because in my research, conversations with my surgeon, and what I have seen from others, it was pretty standard to be admitted after having the SAL surgery. So, now completely overwhelmed, irritated, in pain, blood dripping through my dressings I needed a minute to breathe. The poor guy didn't know what to do because I kept yelling, "STOP," but they heaved me up and *tossed* me to the new bed anyway. My spotlight was over, this move was not fun, and I hated the world.

Then, it occurred to me I needed to use the restroom. My temper flared as my nurse told me I could not get out of bed. She gave me a bowl to use which then caused a heated discussion on whether I could leave the bed or not. By now, I was in fight mode. I was persistent in my demands. I thought that my surgeon wanted me to be up and moving when possible. Despite the dopiness, I vividly remembered this conversation before going under. Needless to say, I lost round one and held it in. I refused to go while sitting in my bed. A few hours later I said to my nurse "Okay I have **got** to go, and I am NOT going in my bed." That's when she looked at my chart and read, reluctantly, that it was specified for me to get out of bed to use the restroom. I have a bit of an insolent side of me, so it took everything in me to not say, "I told you so." I, however, may have said it with my face because my mother gave me "the look." You know, the look you get from your parents as a kid that says, "Don't you dare!" Yeah three kids and thirty-nine years later my mother had very much perfected this look.

It felt like eternity before receiving my milkshake given the uncomfortable state I was in. This operation was overwhelmingly more painful than the year before. The pain in my right leg was so substantial from the SAL that I could hardly tell my left leg had been operated on as well. I really couldn't feel any pain at all in my left leg from the LVA. I had no nausea and, although it was not quite as dry this time, my throat was still very sore. My mom stayed with me as my overnight guest while Dad and Trey went back to the hotel. The morning came, and I was discharged to go.

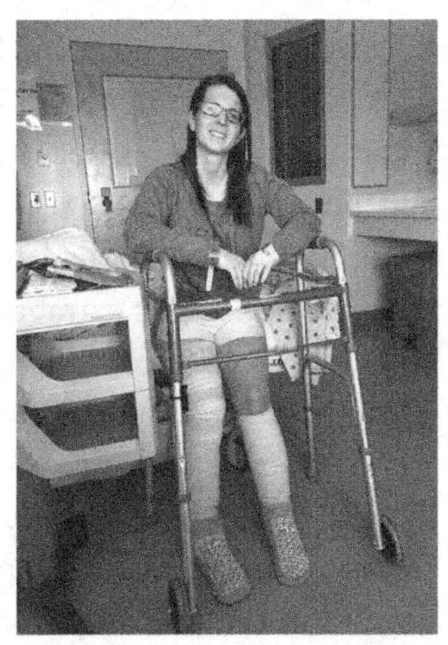

Sitting stagnant in a car after surgery is never comfortable. This time Trey drove me as we followed my parents. Halfway back we made a pit stop for snacks, drinks, and to use the facilities. During the past few hours, my throat, like last time, had been sore and bothering me, but I hadn't quite thought anything of it. After trying to eat a snack, it started to burn. Thinking this slightly unusual, I pulled down the sun visor and looked in the mirror. Much to my surprise, my uvula was completely white. Great, something I didn't think to check before leaving the hospital. I immediately called my primary care physician's office. Thankfully this was on a Thursday. Unfortunately, Dr. M nor FNP JK were available, so they set me up with another colleague in the office who could see me the next day. I was shocked to learn from a swab test that I had developed uvulitis. What is it with me having surgeries on my legs, but having post-op complications in my throat? Looking at the brighter side of things, I found it comical at this point, but it masked the fact it's just so strange. This honestly made recovery terrible, and it wasn't even the area of my body that was cut open. There were very few foods I could eat without a burning sensation.

Over the weekend, Trey and I went out for fresh air and to eat. I ordered a salad and had to be "that difficult customer" who picked apart her food over a simple salad. It was obvious I had undergone an operation—crutches, hospital dressings and hospital socks. I wasn't even wearing shoes. I laughed, apologised and said I had an infected uvula from the tube for the anesthesia. Our extraordinary waitress at the local Italian restaurant set aside any judgement by making sure I had what I could eat. It was a memorable outing during my recovery.

At home I had my recovery kingdom sorted and set up for the coming days. There were pillows, a large water cup, snacks, remotes, and my laptop. My choice of show to binge watch was the Star Wars original series. During this time my family would take turns taking me on what we called little adventures. This was to get me out of the house for some fresh air, but I only had the energy for an hour or so at a time.

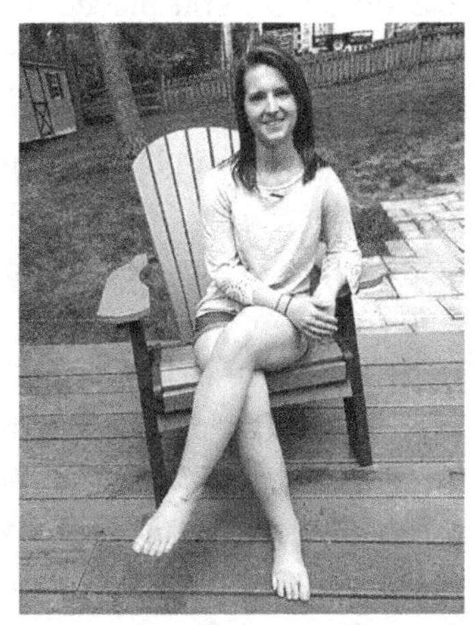

One week later, I had my first post-op appointment. My dad drove me back up to Baltimore. Trips with him are always an adventure. Sitting in the car totaling eight to nine hours in one day really took a toll on the surgical swelling. Healing from trauma made sitting in a stagnant position all day extremely difficult. By the time we got home that evening, my feet were so large and swollen, they really did look like one of the hobbit's feet from Lord of the Rings. I was petrified that they would be like that forever. I was acting so dramatically, it's actually comical to think back on. It's hard to believe what the body can do, but it truly is amazing how the body heals, morphs and shapes itself. My mom assured me they would heal and not be hobbit feet forever. My biggest lesson here is mother always knows best!

Four days later, a strange thing happened. It is only seen once in a lifetime, if then. The country shut down. A virus unknown to humankind swept across the nation, as well as the world, and our governor mandated a stay-at-home policy. I am very lucky and thankful my surgery was taken care of just in time before all this. During the shutdown, the procedure I had was not labeled as a surgery important enough to have for the next year or so. I also had two months to stay at home and focus on healing. I am very sad and sorry for the circumstances of my good fortune, but I do think the time off work and life in general played a huge role on having such a positive outcome. One liter of fluid was removed from my right leg and my left leg was given two new routes for the lymph fluid to flow through the veins. The quality of my life changed drastically.

By now, I was well on my way to accepting this disease. I posted more and more on social media wanting to become more involved. I shared my story, ups and downs with whoever would listen. This is how I virtually met Betty, founder of *Lymphedema Podcast*. She reached out back in 2019, wanting to do an episode on the LVA surgery. I couldn't believe it. I wasn't the first or the only one to have this surgery done, but I was chosen to be a guest pertaining to this topic. For the first time I felt seen. I felt important. Episode 32 "LVA Surgery: Kiersten's Story" turned out to be the number one most listened to episode of 2019 out of forty-five episodes. I couldn't believe it when she made the big reveal a few days shy of the beginning of the new year. Out of so many amazing different topics and guest speakers, people chose to listen to my story the most. I was beyond honoured, grateful, and in disbelief. Someone needed to pinch me because I truly thought I was dreaming.

After Trey and I got married, Betty reached out again about doing another episode. This episode was to discuss Trey's perspective as a lymphoedema spouse. This also involved how we managed the disease during the wedding as well as honeymooning out of the country. My episodes include *Episode 32: Kiersten's Lymphatic Surgery Story*, *2023 Lymphedema Podcast Season 5: Episode 12*, and *2023 Lymphedema Podcast Season 5: Episode 13*.

Speechless

The summer of 2022 was arguably the worst period of the eight years since I had been diagnosed with lymphoedema. My left limb reached its limit; it was unable to function any longer. The swelling increased ferociously. Every step I took became difficult. I avoided stairs as much as possible and every aspect of life was miserable. Whether the change was gradual or overnight, I am not completely sure. All I am sure of is that it felt like it happened in the blink of an eye.

My left foot stretched out like a balloon. I don't just mean that figuratively. I couldn't fit into any footwear anymore. Barn boots? Out of the question. Tennis shoes? They weren't wide enough. Even most of my flip-flops were unwearable. Every step I took was painful and miserable. Birkenstocks became my saving grace. Sitting down was agonising. I could feel my skin stretching thinner and thinner. My left calf wasn't far behind being visibly full and tight with fluid. And the limb was persistently not responding to therapies. It was extremely difficult to avoid thinking now, more than ever, "Why is this happening to me? What have I done to deserve this?" I could no longer walk up a staircase. I used the elevator at work every day. This alone says a lot because I have hated elevators ever since I was a little girl. I have spent my whole life avoiding them because they make me feel sick. Riding my horse was no longer fun and I couldn't fit in my riding boots and chaps—again. My horse—who is my escape, my therapy, my happy place—became a burden to my pain.

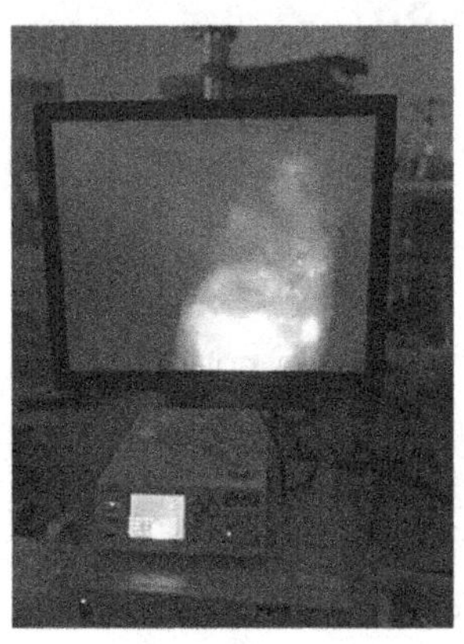

Dr. Aliu

It felt like the universe was conspiring against me. It's one of those things where you can feel on top of the world, conquering the disease, and then you just get completely crushed by it. This is the roller coaster ride lymphoedema famously inflicts on its victims.

This rebellion of my lymphatics decided to come full force, just as my surgeon was moving farther away, leaving me stranded. It would be a few more months until he started at a new hospital and then I would have to find the right office to make an appointment. When September came, I could finally get on his schedule. In the meantime, the mental weight took a step back into despair and grief. I grieved the loss of normality.

When I finally saw Dr. Aliu, he agreed something needed to be done for my left leg. Although I had already undergone LVA for this limb, my insurance company required I try it again before considering the more invasive approach, the LNT. Also, at the new hospital Dr. Aliu did not have access to the lymphography test in the office as he did in Maryland. The equipment was only located in the operating room. So, the lymphography test and preparations for LVA surgery were scheduled for October. As frustrating as it was to go through this process because of insurance, I am extremely grateful to have a surgeon I could go to with my concerns.

A month later, I woke up in the outpatient room. My toes were green—from the pigment of the injected dye—, my skin clean, exposed to the air, and my surgeon by my side. He began the procedure with the lymphography test, only to find out that at this point the lymphatic channels were completely shot.

I was devastated, desperate for relief, and in tears.

(In saying that, I want to make a point to note that I was not upset nor disappointed with my surgeon nor by the decision he made. I have the highest regard for my surgeon's professional judgement; therefore, I trust him implicitly with my care. We already had a plan B in place, which he was very optimistic about. The only challenge would be insurance. Trey and I had traveled to Pennsylvania from Virginia for this. It is about an eight-hour drive (depending on stops). We had made it an overnight trip, only to end up going home the same as I was the day before. What I have had to learn and understand about lymphoedema is that, because of the resources available, I sometimes just don't know the extent of the condition until after trips are booked, money is paid, and anesthesia is administered.)

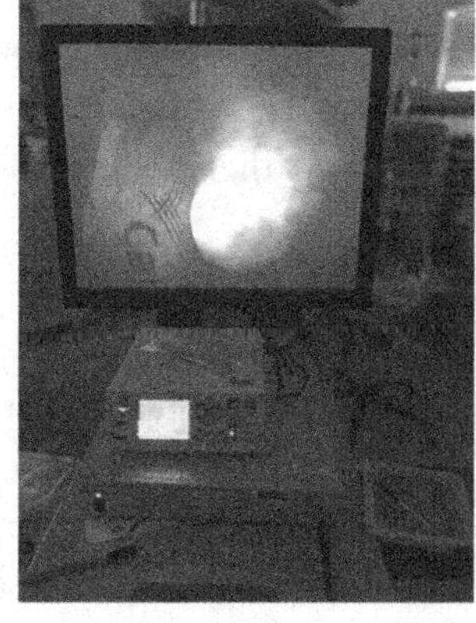

Dr. Aliu

My left leg had deteriorated significantly over the previous six months, and the lymphatic channels were no longer intact. There was fluid everywhere. There is no reason or explanation for this, other than the fact that my lifestyle was simply paired with a malfunctioning lymphatic system. These are the cards I was dealt, and I have to take extra care of myself. So, we planned to schedule the LNT from the omentum to left leg as well as SAL in the left leg and foot.

With lymphoedema, I have learned you have got to find the good things that come out of it. So, what did I get out of this short trip? I got the answers I had been wanting all summer. I was able to see the internal damage. I had a fun two days traveling with my best friend. I finally got to meet a lipo-lymphoedema friend in person. I found a local candy shop that had my favourite childhood candy, which I used to buy in England. Lastly, for breakfast, we got these amazing little doughnuts even though I couldn't swallow them due to a dry throat.

Life went on and things were being put in motion to schedule surgery for the LNT and SAL in my left lower quadrant with Dr. Aliu, as well as a general surgeon. Unfortunately, insurance was bound and determined to not allow this surgery to happen, but they didn't know who they were messing with. I *would* fight back.

The first claim put in for surgery came back denied. Their reason (and their most frequent excuse) was "we don't cover cosmetic procedures." Anyone who suffers from this disease knows it is absolutely not a cosmetic issue. It is the loss of function of a system in the body that regulates lymphatic fluid. This is a disease not a cosmetic blemish. So, we appealed. Oh, and for the sake of a time frame, this started in October 2022. The claim came back denied, once again stating that it's cosmetic: "Your doctor ordered a procedure to remove fat under the skin…" This really gets my blood boiling inside because that is not what is being ordered. This is how the insurance companies want to interpret the claims to avoid paying the cost. I was 4'11" and weighed no more than 110 pounds; I didn't have any fat to remove. The next step was a peer-to-peer review. This is when your surgeon speaks with an insurance approved doctor to determine whether surgery is medically necessary. In other words, a doctor who knows nothing about you and has never seen you is now determining the necessity of your medical needs. The fact that this is legal is mind-blowing to me. Also, the peer-to-peer review **must** be done prior to the operation (I learned this the hard way with my first surgery in 2019). After the consultation, the insurance's doctor stuck to their denials and refused to approve the surgery. Again, someone who knew nothing about me was making critical life decisions that would affect my body, my way of living, and my quality of life.

To keep this story simple regarding the back and forth battle I went through, I appealed six times prior to the day of surgery: December 13, 2022. The insurance company denied five of those appeals deeming the surgery to be "cosmetic." (It's not cosmetic). The sixth appeal, five days prior to surgery date, was when they decided that the portion of the surgery that the general surgeon was performing was not covered simply because the plan did not cover it.

When it comes to this process, one has to understand there are many parts to a procedure that may or may not be covered. In addition, there are lots of moving parts in the claims process. So, this denial was disappointing to hear, but for that specific aspect of the surgery, it was what it was. They weren't calling it cosmetic nor experimental, I just had really inadequate insurance at the time. But the week before surgery, there was still no approval for Dr. Aliu's role in the procedure. We chose to stay the course and the hospital filed one more appeal, labeling it as urgent considering surgery was only a few business days away, in order to try to push this through for my sake.

Finally, it was Sunday, December 11, 2022. Mom, Trey, and I drove up to Pittsburgh, Pennsylvania a couple days early due to inclement weather showing on the radar. We had the most amazing pizza for dinner! We sat down in the basement of a restaurant in the city enjoying the evening despite the cold, snowy weather. I had an Airbnb booked for the next day through my first post-op appointment ten days later.

On Monday, December 12th we were getting ready to start our day and prepare for the recovery to come. At 9:30am, I was in my mom's hotel room watching the weather when my phone rang with the hospital's caller ID. I answered excitedly, expecting this to be the phone call from the operating room (OR) scheduler telling me what time I needed to arrive the next morning. To my despair, this was not the case. It was one of the nurses in the hospital's office calling to tell me the surgery had been canceled due to no final response from insurance. I quickly put the phone on speaker just to have another set of ears listen to the conversation. I didn't do this with the intent of my parent to chime in. My mom knows I'm an adult and gave me the opportunity to handle it while silently listening in awe. I lack confidence when it came to phone calls which is why I prefer to have a second set of ears for important conversations such as this. I think I had a solid ten seconds of silence to consider whether I heard her correctly. I was completely caught off guard and basically my response was "no", I will not stand for this. I will not allow insurance to dictate my life. I will not allow insurance to dictate what I can and can't do nor the medical care I can and can't have. She was just the messenger, so I tried really hard to keep myself composed and to honestly not break into tears. I explained I was upset to hear this when I wasn't even consulted. It sounded like it was done and telling me was an afterthought. I, hopefully nicely, demanded to be put back on the schedule. I was having surgery. Between the hotel rooms for one night, food on the road, gas and the Airbnb, there was already $2,000 invested in this surgery that we couldn't get back. Not to mention the hoops I had to jump through for my six-week short term disability from work. It was all just more collateral damage that comes with this disease. We were there, I was in pain, and this was going to happen. Not to mention it was two surgeons we had to coordinate schedules with. I expressed clearly that I understood I was choosing to go into a costly surgery without any help from insurance and that fighting the denial would be much more difficult after the operation was completed. I was willing to go through a tougher battle. I was ready. We peacefully got off the phone with the plan to stay the course. She called back thirty minutes later confirming everyone was still on board, and I would be receiving a phone call from someone to discuss the financial side of it as well as still needing the phone call from the OR scheduler.

What was supposed to be the most exciting day of the year became the most nerve-wracking. I know we left the phone call that morning with the plan to stay the course, but I just didn't feel good about it until I could hear from a scheduler. We stuck around the hotel a little longer, flabbergasted at what just happened. We needed a minute to let it sink in.

That afternoon we found the Airbnb and got all settled. It wasn't your fancy rental home, but, despite a few freaky pieces of artwork, it was cheap and provided exactly what we needed to function. We familiarised ourselves with where everything was since that would be home for a while. We also took some time to drive around the area. By the end of our trip, it really did feel like we lived there.

Mid-afternoon came around and still nothing from the hospital. We decided to keep going as if nothing ever happened. Mom and I went to the grocery store while Trey was getting in some final meetings uninterrupted. Finally, my phone rang nice and loud. It was the scheduler! Of course, with my luck, she called during the one time of the day I was out in public and had to answer personal questions. Ironically, I found solace in the beer aisle and was able to get my arrival time as well as go through the rest of the information needed to prepare for a procedure. Mom continued to shop around, despite her excitement, but stayed close by in case I needed anything. At last, I let out a huge breath of relief.

On the way back to the house, my phone rang again. This time it was someone to discuss the transparency of the cost without insurance. Due to the mountainous terrain of Pittsburgh, the phone service would quickly go in and out. Mom pulled over in a neighborhood when we hit a clear spot. This conversation sucked. I one hundred percent understood what I was getting myself into, but it's a whole different feeling when you actually hear the numbers. Potentially, I was getting myself into a five-figure medical debt. And I say potentially only because I was going to continue to fight tooth and nail for insurance to pay their fair share. This was at four in the afternoon, and the offices closed at five. We got off the phone and were staying the course.

This was the first time I think I finally looked at my mom. There were tears in her eyes. She was worried I wouldn't be able to walk down the aisle on my wedding day. She said to me, "Health is more important than a dollar sign." We had a really emotional talk, but ultimately, insurance or no insurance, the surgery *had* to happen. Back at the house, I updated Trey. Everything was confirmed. Without insurance backing me up, we would be heading to the hospital at five in the morning on Tuesday, December 13, 2022.

Sixteen Hours

December 14, 2022
Pittsburgh, Pennsylvania

I truly don't know how to describe what it was like when I woke up. I was more dazed and confused than I had been in the past. I was just cut open with twenty incisions from my abdomen to my toes. Pain was a given, but my arm hurt even more. My eyes were swollen shut. I asked myself, "What have I done?"

I woke up, but something was strange; something was different. I was in excruciating pain. However, my throat wasn't dry, nor was it sore. My throat had always been my biggest problem waking up from anesthesia. But this time, my throat didn't hurt a bit. My leg was definitely on fire and I thought I was going to die, my typical dramatic reaction. By now, a nurse walking by had noticed me stirring and called for my assigned nurse. He was at my bedside checking vitals within seconds. I could hardly open my eyes. My arms were significantly swollen and burning with pain. Despite my complaints, my nurse didn't know how to help. My left arm was not involved in the surgery, so there was nothing to explain the pain. There were no visible signs of a medical issue. It was later decided that my arm could have been placed in an unnatural position throughout the operation. This may have caused the pain when my arm returned to a normal position for the blood flow. Before I was put under, I was told the operation was expected to take eight hours putting it around dinner time when completed. In saying this, my next thought was "I am STARVING." I had never felt hunger so desperately in my life. Extremely dramatic, I know. Saying I had an empty stomach was an understatement. I gurgled out halfway incoherently, "Have I missed dinner? When can I eat?" My nurse turned to me, and despite being blind as a bat without my glasses I could feel the baffled look, and he stated, "Dinner? It's almost breakfast." I processed this for a second. I cautiously asked, "What DAY is it?" "It's Wednesday. It's 3:15 in the morning. Your surgery took 16 hours. Your family is still in the waiting area."

Because there were no nurses on duty and the length of the operation, it took longer than usual for someone to be able to find my personal belongings. When it was determined I was okay, they wheeled me out of ICU to the hospital room prepared for me. That would be "home" for the next two full days. It was still early in the morning, so my first nurse was the overnight nurse who still had a couple hours left of her shift. She was so nice and such a saint! I wish I could have had the opportunity to thank her for dealing with me. I know there were times I was likely rude, but being in that amount of pain, it was very difficult for my brain to have that awareness. During this time, everything was just plain frustrating.

I physically needed help with every movement. I wasn't allowed to use my abdomen muscles for a month. When I

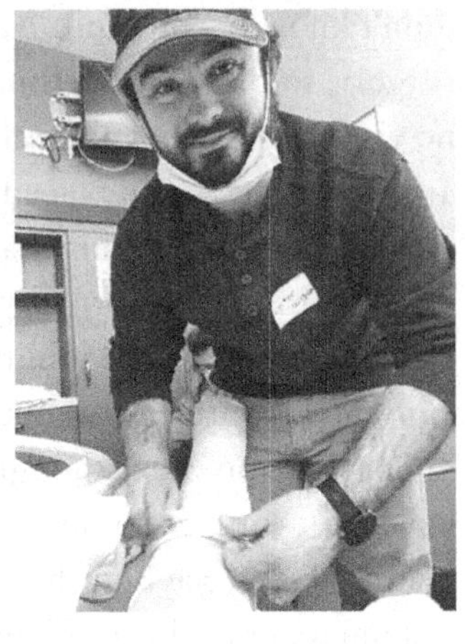

wanted to sit up someone had to push my back forward and readjust the pillows. I had never been so uncomfortable in my life. We had *everything* elevated. My body was so filled with fluids. Trey would freshen the bandages on my right leg each day managing this leg during the time that I couldn't. Sheets had to be changed every few hours or so from the three drains I had in my left leg. It was a very dirty time. I already couldn't wait until my first shower.

I was on a broth-only diet for a while. They allowed jello as well, but I didn't like the flavours they had available. So, I stuck with water and chicken broth for 36 hours. I took hangry to a whole new level during this time.

The nights were the most difficult. Unfortunately, there were not enough nurses to patients. Visitors not being allowed during these hours made it very difficult to stay on top of medicine. I would call for help when I needed to use the restroom or have the next dose of medicine and a nurse would not show for 15, 20, or even 30 minutes at a time. There was one occasion I started crying in pain. A nurse heard me and asked why I hadn't called in the remote. I told her I had 25 minutes ago and still no one had come. (I don't mention this to throw the hospital nor their team under the bus. I mention it simply because it was part of my journey and this time admitted in the hospital.) One of the nurses even took the time to listen to a brief conversation on my story and I showed her my lymphoedema Instagram page. That made me incredibly happy and I forgot about the pain for just a few minutes. During a bathroom trip in the night, I had to go so bad I was rushing with my crutch, tripped and fell right as the nurse stepped back to give me some privacy. I fell on the sink hitting about half the incisions on my body. My oversized gown fell off my shoulders and all modesty went completely out the window. I didn't care at that point.

The days were boring and gruesome. It moved slowly for everyone trying to help get my mind off the pain. We talked about what we would eat for the next week and some places around town we would give a try. I messaged a few locals I knew for recommendations.

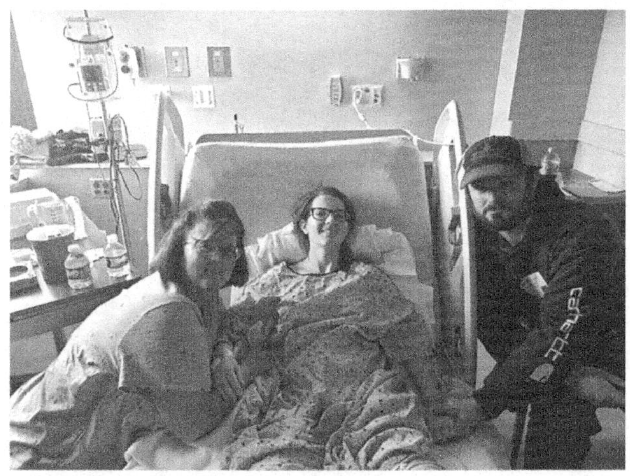

That Thursday afternoon an orthopedic doctor and a few of his students and nurses visited me for an evaluation. They did some movements and checked for any pain outside of the obvious. They cleared my physical well-being to leave the hospital at this point post-surgery. Both the orthopedic doctor as well as Dr. Aliu left it up to me on whether I stayed or was discharged. At the time, I still hadn't had any food, was draining excess fluid, and I required too much help to get up to use the bathroom. I looked at the entrance of the room and the thought of moving farther than that doorway, for the first time, gave me an ill feeling. I decided to stay through one more night. This proved the right decision when the following day I was in much higher spirits to relocate.

Finally, for dinner on Thursday I could eat real, solid food. My first meal since Monday evening. We chose Chipotle! And yes, upon delivery from Trey there ensued a meltdown. Emotions were through the roof during these few days! But we got it fixed and I ate *all* of my burrito bowl over the next several hours.

The Biggest Challenge of All

The time Trey, my mom, and I spent on that trip have become some of my fondest memories. The only unfortunate feature of the house was the number of stairs it had. Because of the hilly region of Pittsburgh, the houses were tall and skinny. Once I was discharged from the hospital, going up a whole flight of fifteen stairs was not an option. Thank God Trey was with us because my mother, bless her, would not have been able to help me in and out of the house. Now, the hospital did offer in-care nurse assistance, but since we had an able-bodied young person with us, we opted out of the in-home care to save a little money. Getting out of the car was a show in itself. It wasn't easy the first time, but we eventually figured out the best approach: one person would pull me from behind while the other gently supported my legs while they were lowered. As I mentioned, however, the first time was not pretty. Plus, we had to watch out for bits of ice on the ground. Trey practically carried me all the way around the house to the back through the kitchen door. This entrance had just three steps to enter the house, making it far more accessible than the front door. In contrast, entering through the front meant stepping into the basement and then climbing a fifteen-step staircase to reach the main floor. But first, we had to get through the icy death trap of the sidewalk.

A few nights prior to my arrival, wrapped as a mummy in a hospital gown, my organised and prepared self already had my kingdom set up. The sofa bed was out, my side table in place, a book, colouring books, and stuffed animals for squeezing out the pain were all set in place. Now all I had to worry about was keeping up with my need for water, snacks, and meals. My alarm clock was set to go off every two hours for medicine. The pain was immeasurable; because of the severe bruising, no position was comfortable. I just had to endure it. The weight of gravity pulling down my limb every time I had to get up was agonizing. I had to move slowly in small increments putting my leg partially down, bringing it back up, then repeating the process moving it further along each time until I was on my feet. Teams A and B took turns gently pushing from behind to help me sit-up because I could not use my core muscles. This process is indescribable, but overall the surgery was well worth everything I endured. The medicine was staggered between Acetaminophen and a prescribed narcotic. The alarms helped me to stay ahead of the pain and stay on track with taking the medication at safe intervals. My mom, from whom I get my organizational skills, created a shared Google Doc between the three of us. Whenever I took medicine, it was recorded by who provided it to me. This also helped alleviate any potential confusion about what I had and when. This continued for weeks—all day and all night. It didn't really hinder any sleep at night because I had literally all day to do nothing. So, I was snoozing on and off, simply because I was so tired. Also, if I could fall asleep, it helped to relieve the pain. It's funny though—despite the pain I was in, I not only slept, but I slept well. And I slept a lot.

There was a constant laundry cycle going to clean dressings and blankets as well as regular replacement of pads used for the blood and fluid coming from the drains. We had a system and as my husband puts it, "This is the most Kiersten thing I've ever seen." I can't help but say I get it from my mother. The nights quickly became lonely. In the hospital, I was allowed visitors only during the day. When I was discharged, I didn't want to disturb Mom and Trey, so they could get some quality sleep. I know being a caretaker is exhausting work. As cranky and harsh as I was in the beginning, I tried my best to be reasonable when I could. Thanks to our fabulous, positive, lymphoedema community, I found that a lymphoedema friend also had the liposuction surgery the same day. We had each other for company, and I didn't feel so lonely. Especially at night when we couldn't sleep but could share the pain and experience and understand what the other was going through. I enjoyed our conversations over Instagram and the connection we had.

The next day, it started to snow. This was on Saturday, my first full day moved into the Airbnb. I probably hadn't seen snow in December since I was a child. You would have thought I was a little girl again because I was so excited. I just stared out the window for hours watching each unique ice crystal fall from the sky. Despite the pain, I enjoyed that day very much. The snow stopped and I curled back into my dungeon under the covers and continued with many appeals for assistance.

A few more days passed by and I woke up to just another normal day with the same routine. It was first thing in the morning and my husband was up making breakfast before he had to log into his morning meetings. To my astonishment, he joked that I was living in a dungeon, walked over to the windows next to me, and threw open the blinds. It was like a scene from a movie. I nearly shrieked at the bright light that suddenly hit my eyes. I was grumpy, hungry, and had just woken up to an alarm an hour prior. He demanded I get some sunlight, even if it was just coming through the window. I wasn't ready to sit up for the day, but considering I was immobile, I didn't have a choice; he proceeded to prop me up. It was for the better. I was taking advantage of this time to be lazy without any responsibilities.

Five days after surgery, the time came. My first bowel movement. I had learned my lesson in the past, so I had been preparing for this moment by drinking a ton of water, taking stool softener, and eating foods containing fiber. From my experience, this event was arguably worse than the surgery. It's in that moment that things start to move, but it's not quite there yet. So, trying to find some sense of humor to lighten the situation, I made an Instagram reel making my way to the bathroom to Rafiki from the Lion King around the, "it is time" moment. I thought it was pretty funny and my followers got a good kick out of it as well. It didn't take too long for there to be no humor in the situation. I was *screaming* in pain. I was not supposed to be using those muscles. To be honest, I am surprised I didn't pop open any incisions. It's a very difficult situation for your caretaker (or caretakers in my case) to help because there really isn't anything they can do. It was a Sunday, but we did have a number to call for nurses in case we needed anything. Between mom making phone calls and Trey taking a trip or two to the local Walgreens, relief finally came after six hours of pushing. I nearly passed out from all the excessive strain. Finally, the worst part of the surgery had passed.

Unfortunately, not everyone in this world receives three meals a day. There is hunger and starvation among many communities in all countries. This surgery has given me so much more awareness to the difference in meaning between "I am hungry," versus "I am starving." After being out for so long and on a broth only diet for a couple more days, I had never experienced pure hunger like I did after this surgery. When I was given the okay to eat solid food, my first meal was Chipotle. I had to eat in stages because of the feeling I got having food in my stomach again. I was also terrified knowing the constipation would be coming. It took a week for my stomach to finally feel full again. I have always used the phrase "I'm starving," when I have been super hungry. I will never use this phrase again because there are people in this world who are genuinely starving. I am blessed to have food on the table each day. Others may not be as lucky.

Lymphoedema has taught me to be grateful for what I have. It has taught me to be a kinder person and not take life for granted.

Recovery's Battlefield

The drive back to Virginia was brutal. My husband and my mom packed the cars, cleaned the house, then prepared to move me. I began "walking" from the back door—because remember, the front door had a whole flight of stairs involved—to the car. It was slow, exhausting, and painful, but we got there. To get in the truck, I leaned against the back seat and from the other side my husband pulled me in from behind while my mom was supporting my legs from the front. I can imagine this was quite the scene, but it was effective and kept me from hitting my drains or sensitive areas. I was so tucked in with pillows and blankets, I was as snug as a bug. With my leftovers in hand and ready to fall asleep, we said bye to the strange little house that had been home.

Starting the drive, I was curious to know what it was like for Trey and my mom (Michele) during the later hours of the surgery. "Around 2 a.m., Dr. Aliu came into the waiting room with a long-drawn face and looked extremely tired. Mrs. Michele started crying. He perked up and let us know all was well and what happened. He then said to hang out and a nurse would come get us." Trey continued, "Well, the office assistant had left for the evening the day before and came

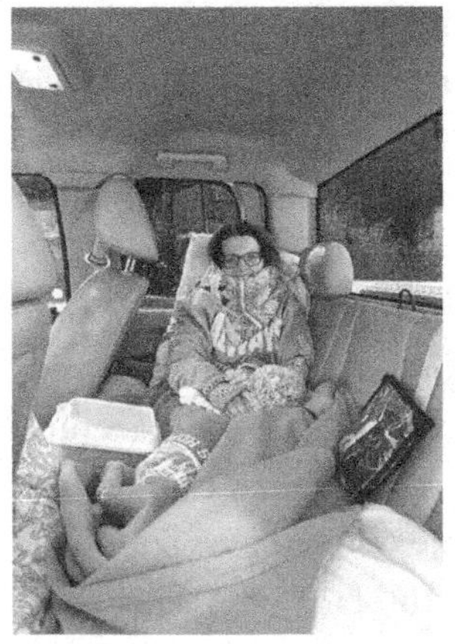

back for her next day of work to find us still there in the waiting room. When she realised we had been there all night, she perked up and said, 'Come along, I'll help you find her. I'm sorry.' She found your room and sent us there. We were going to beat you there, but we actually saw you being rolled in right before we got there. Mrs. Michele burst crying again when she saw you and you were crying because your arms were swollen and you thought you now had lymphoedema in your arms." I thought the whole thing was crazy. I was under for *sixteen hours*, but it truly felt like I had blinked.

After light conversation, I slept for most of the drive. We made plans to make a pit stop at my godparents' house for the night to give me a break from the car and a nice home cooked meal. By this point, we were within the borders of Virginia and only a couple hours away from home. That night was the first time I was allowed to finally take a full-blown shower instead of just a sponge bath. This was the most glorious shower I have ever had. My godmother's bathroom had just been renovated and it was on the ground level where I slept. With only three steps to conquer getting into the house, it was a very convenient set-up. Only a few steps from the bathroom was the recliner that became my spot for the next twelve hours. I made myself comfortable, got my feet propped up, and simply soaked in the moment, feeling as fresh as a warm spring day.

I remember we had spaghetti and garlic bread that night. My appetite was still monumental, so I devoured every bite.

After dinner we enjoyed one another's company. We talked about wedding planning, and the surgery. My godparents had their young dog put up knowing that her energy would be too much around my weak physical state. However, their older beagle, Cassie, was in our presence. While we were talking, no one noticed Cassie walking to the front of my chair to plop herself in her favourite spot; someone's lap—mine. In mid-flight, as she jumped up, everyone yelled, "NO!" I gracefully shrieked, bracing for impact. Poor Cassie landed ever so tenderly between my legs not hurting me one bit. Her poor little ears fell back, looking around with the face of, "What did I do?" It makes me giggle thinking about it now.

The evening of the thirteenth day was the hardest. This one was designed to be a crucible. Trey and I traveled to his family's coast house in North Carolina which was a four-hour drive. I was comfortable enough in the back seat of the truck, but you can only be but so comfortable recovering from this procedure. Thankfully, I fell asleep for the whole ride through any jolts of pain. Unfortunately, we did the drive during the late afternoon-early evening; a recipe for not being tired enough to sleep during the night. Sure enough, there I was at 1:18 in the morning, tired, but not that drowsiness kind of tired to be able to fall asleep. The jolts of pain wouldn't stop dancing in my ankle, foot and toes. It honestly felt so much better standing up walking around than it did to be sitting or lying down with my leg elevated. The incisions on my abdomen were also driving me crazy with the itchiness. I took my last narcotic an hour prior and it was slow to take effect. So, there I was sitting up in bed silently burdening the pain. As much as I'd rather avoid staring at a blue-light screen in the dark, it also wouldn't do me any good staring at the ceiling withering away with the weight of the pain on my mind. I channeled my thoughts into writing this book as a way to find a temporary escape from my wounds.

The next thirty-six hours proved to be the most agonizing pain thus far in my life. The nerves in my foot began to wake up with a fierce determination to wreak havoc. It then came to my mind I wasn't put on nerve medication from the beginning like I had been in the past. It was a different hospital, so maybe they had different procedures? In the future, if I have any more operations, I will learn from this lesson. I was desperate for anything to help relieve the pain. I sent an urgent message to my nurses and surgeon. They asked for the nearest pharmacy to send a prescription. So, there we were, on a Friday afternoon the day before a holiday trucking down the road forty minutes away to the nearest pharmacy. I was absolutely useless, completely reliant on my crutches, and in moaning pain. I'm sure I was quite the sight to see.

We waited our turn in line. I am getting stared at but that's a completely normal occurrence by now. Why is it so stare worthy being bandaged and hunched over in pain on crutches? Anyway, we got to the counter and the pharmacist says insurance won't let them fill it because it's not due yet for a refill. I'm starting to feel my temper rising. My short fuse has been lit. Time is ticking away. I told him there is no refill, it was just prescribed an hour ago. I was there to pick it up for the first time. He said there was nothing he could do to help and "didn't know what to tell us." I said, "Fine, I'll call **MY** pharmacist" and stepped aside. (I really can't make this stuff up. My insurance sagas are a piece of work on their own. You couldn't script the nightmares I have faced if you had tried.

When it comes to the pharmacy thank God I have pharmacists in the family.) After letting my brother know what was going on he got frustrated that we weren't helped efficiently. He explained what the problem must have been and gave me a list of steps to go through and then to call him back.

Step one was to ask the nurses where the prescription was sent to. That's when we found out that the online portal sent it to the hospital I was admitted to two weeks prior in Pennsylvania. This explains why I had trouble at the counter. Step two, this was a pain, call the hospital pharmacy to "put the medicine back" and send back the prescription. Do you know how many phone numbers and extensions a hospital has? A lot. After a hot minute of phone calls and transfers I soon got to the correct line. I must have caught the receiver on a bad day because she was way more defensive than necessary. Still keep in mind how much jolting, stabbing pain I am in and now on my feet longer than I had intended. Step three, I let the nurses know I had done my part and they resent the prescription to the pharmacy I was waiting at in North Carolina. Step four, updating my brother. We were getting closer. Here we go again back in line. We get to the counter and explained the steps I had just taken. The pharmacist said he could see the prescription now, but they were about to go on their meal break. He notified me that when they got back it would take about an hour to fill. Joy to the world to the twenty-eight-year-old who wants to fall over dying. I know, I was being dramatic. So, I sat on the floor of the convenience store for ten minutes because my legs and my brain just couldn't hold myself up anymore. Did I tell you this also all happened on a Friday that was New Year's Eve? In essence, though they were normally open, the next day they were going to be closed. It was way too stressful of an afternoon. After coming to the realization that I do have some slight dignity left, Trey and I went next door to Walmart to get a few things. We waited an hour and a half then happily picked up the medication for the nerve pain.

The sad truth of the story is the delay in receiving the medication meant it was unable to provide substantial relief. It helped just enough to be worth taking, but I still couldn't sleep nor was I comfortable for weeks.

The unseen burden of this disease is the weight it causes within. The mental pain, the emotional pain, the financial pain, as well as the physical pain. What others could not see nor feel during this recovery was the feeling every time I put my left leg down. The rushing forces of all fluid and blood being dragged down by gravity. It was a heavy burden to hold amongst my own body. I couldn't just get up in one motion. I had to gradually put my leg down a little bit at a time with intervals of putting it back up before I could start scooting away.

On the eighteenth week of recovery, I was still bandaged for a large part of each day. My flat knit compression garment wasn't comfortable to be in unless I was moving. Plus, my leg was so much smaller than what my garments had been made for the year before. In result, I noticed a lot of increased swelling due to the garment's measurements produced for a larger limb. My left leg was driving me up a wall for a few weeks. It was nerve pain alright, but it wasn't unbearable torture all night long like it had been week three. The pain would come in spurts. The nerves and skin were pissed off to the moon, so it was going to take a long time to heal one hundred percent (as was discussed with me beforehand). What I was experiencing wasn't terrible, but it did still affect my sleep and cause much discomfort during the day.

Six months and five days out sleep was getting better, but still was occasionally affected. The nerves would have a party in my foot once or twice a week. My newest discovery was the recovery of physical activity. I didn't feel like I had a twenty-pound weight strapped to each ankle like I did before. I didn't feel as rushed to get in bandages and I was capable of doing more. In fact, I felt like I had the energy of my 16-year-old self again!

Continuing into 2023, life felt normal for the first time in ten years. Day-to-day activities or obligations were manageable as opposed to impossible. In addition, my mental health flourished. Whenever I was having a tough day, I noticed I stopped blaming my legs for it. Granted, I was still extremely diligent sticking to my complete decongestive therapy regimen. I see some Lymphies only do CDT a few times a year for a few weeks at a time. If that works for you then that's great! However, I find my lymphoedema at its happiest when I am constantly performing CDT. I don't have night garments anymore because I only bandage at night. Again, another trial-and-error tool I discovered to further accommodate the swelling. I dry-brush my skin every day—which also helps with the itches—moisturize, exercise, elevate, and utilize my pneumatic compression pump several times a week for MLD. This is all incorporated into my daily routine. It's hard work,

I won't hide nor deny that. But it is well worth it. Once I got past my grief and denial, I realised *that I need to do what I can today to make it a better tomorrow.* With that mindset it sets me up for success instead of failure.

Well, by the summer I was feeling more and more disconnected from racing. I absolutely loved my boss and appreciated the experience I was gaining. But I was no longer happy in this role. I wanted to be more directly involved with the horses and horsemen.

So, I called my old boss from the farm that I can never seem to get away from. Eagle Point Farm will always have a special place in my heart. I asked the trainer if she needed any extra help on the backside of the racetrack. I dearly missed taking care of horses. Since my legs were doing significantly better, I felt capable to take on part-time hours for the couple months of the season. We agreed on twelve hours a week and it was a blast! One more thing I can check-off my dream list; working as a groom and hot-walker at a racetrack. It's such a different environment and a thrilling feeling. I didn't do this because I needed the extra money (although I did use the money for myself and purchased something I had been wanting for a very long time). I did it for the love of the horses and for racing. I love the quick pace environment. There's nothing better than a well-oiled shed row. It was exhausting waking up at four every morning, getting in two hours of hard labour, showering in the bath house, then changing for my eight-hour shift for my clerical job. Then after that I had my own horse to ride and responsibilities at his barn to fulfill.

The fact that I could complete this made my heart so happy. Once the racing season ended, I was exhausted, a little more fit, and slightly glad it was over. However, every second of it was worth it for the fun I had for those two hours each day. The accomplishment I felt for my lymphoedema holding up through all this shows me how far I have come. Lastly, rewarding myself with a brand new, beautiful dressage saddle left me bursting with emotions. It was the newest model on the market for the brand I chose. Summer of 2023 left me over the moon with joy for the journey I had taken.

October came around and working the horse sales became even more enjoyable. I sure do have a story to share with you! Working the sales, we are required to wear khaki pants or shorts. I found it very difficult to find either that fit my figure and swelling in a lady-like and appropriate way. Back in 2020 I had gotten several pairs from American Eagle after a suggestion from a friend; thanks Megan! They were bootcut and a stretchy material. The perfect combination for a Lymphie! They served their purpose for a few seasons. The week of the 2022 October horse sale I took them out of storage and, due to the increased swelling of my left leg, I had to force, squeeze, and shimmy to get them on. It was terribly uncomfortable and they were just way too tight on my legs. It made my already popping out attributes pop out even more. It was too late to try to find new pairs, so I sucked it up and wore them for the four days of the sale alternating days with shorts. Well, in September of 2023, nine months after my LNT, I took them out again weeks in advance to give myself time to buy new khakis. I was so excited to have a reason to buy new pants since they did not fit the year before. Well, I put them on and because of the surgery the darn things fit even better than they did when I had originally bought them! Who would've thought I would have actually been sad to fit in a pair of pants with lymphoedema? I kept the pants, but I still went to Bass Pro Shop anyway and found two new pairs to take to the sale. They had lots of pockets and working with horses we love pockets!

Upon arriving the night before the first day, one of my friends was also pulling in the parking lot of the hotel. This is the only time of the year I see these friends, so I excitedly hollered her name. The last time she had seen me was a year prior, swollen and struggling to function. I ran to her with bandages and all. She stopped dead in her tracks flabbergasted at what she saw. She was beyond ecstatic for the mobility I got back thanks to the surgery. Even though she lived across the country, she followed and supported my story every step of the way. Everyone in my life is so cognizant and supportive, it truly gets me through each day.

Throughout my twenties, I felt I needed to work multiple jobs because I just wasn't making enough money to pay the bills. Because of the lymphoedema I was having a really hard time figuring out what I wanted to do with my life. I originally wanted to be a jockey, but that had to change. Then, I wanted to be a groom; however, that had to change too. The lymphoedema prevented me from physically being capable of riding racehorses or being a groom. Finally, I got my foot in the door at Colonial Downs Racetrack as a seasonal assistant to racing. From there I found full-time employment as the Payroll Clerk in 2021. At last, a solid, full-time job that contributed to paying the bills, was associated with the Thoroughbred industry, and accommodated my chronic swelling.

Recovery (of the LNT) was long, brutal, and exhausting, but every second of it was so worth going through the surgery.

Recovery wasn't only about physically recovering from the surgical trauma to my body. Recovering also meant channeling the little energy I had to focus on not only winning the battle, but also winning the war with insurance.

Fighting an insurance claim is not a joke. If any of my care were to be denied simply because my insurance plan wasn't in a tier that would cover the claim, then that's a whole different course. However, to tell me my claim was denied because it was "not medically necessary" for my debilitating disease that affects my ability to walk is completely unacceptable.

The process I went through to get justice for my most recent surgery in 2022 was pure hell. The best advice I can provide is to stay organised and keep detailed notes of **everything**. The journey began, as I explained earlier, when Dr. Aliu needed to try the LVA again in my left leg in the fall of 2022. This was to check the box for insurance to say we tried a less invasive method and confirmed it was not the right, nor successful, course of action. The next step was sending in a claim for the LNT and SAL scheduled for a few months later in December. On November 7, 2022, I received a letter in the mail from the insurance company (who I shall not name) stating, "Denied for Suction Assisted Lipectomy Lower Extremity and Free Fascial Flap with Microvascular Anastomosis. Purpose: '…your doctor ordered a procedure to remove fat from under your skin… The information we have does not show that the criteria has been met. For this reason, this request is denied as cosmetic.'" I think most patients crumble at these denials and say, "it is what it is." **Never crumble!** Never fold or succumb to their refusals! If we all stand together, we can make a difference. So, with this, I appealed the claim and my surgeon requested a peer-to-peer review.

On November 11, 2022 another letter from insurance came in the mail as a separate piece from the first. The LNT requires at least one day in the hospital so, the denial read as follows, "Denied for 1-day hospital stay. Purpose: '...your doctor ordered a procedure to remove fat from under your skin... The information we have does not show that the criteria has been met. For this reason, this request is denied as cosmetic.'" What are the criteria you may ask? As listed in the letter: "1. The person has a problem with normal functioning or infections." I could not fit into clothing nor walk up a flight of stairs any longer. So, clearly the criteria was met. "2. This procedure is expected to improve functioning." Having full mobility of my leg for the first time in several years? That's a given. "3. The person has not been helped by other treatment that has been tried for at least 3 months (for example, compression garments and other treatments)." I had not just three months worth, but four years' worth of proof that treatment had not helped. Two months prior we also tried the LVA which did not help. And lastly, "4. After the procedure is done, the person will continue with other treatment (compression garments and other treatments)." I don't understand how this could be included because it is not something that can be predicted prior to surgery, but given my history I would clearly meet this criteria. So, as far as myself and my entire medical team were concerned, all the criteria were met. However, some person sitting behind a desk who had no idea who I was or knew anything about me decided, for some reason, I had not met the criteria and therefore denied this life saving procedure.

It was only five days later when I received the next denial in the mail. "Denied for surgical stay in hospital. Purpose: 'Your plan doesn't cover care that's Cosmetic.'" Despite continuing the appeal, on December 5th and December 6th

of 2022 I received letters stating the same purpose for the denial—that my claim was cosmetic. However, the surgery had nothing to do with visual attributes nor any fat in my body. The last denial, before the operation, came the week before on December 9th denying the general surgeon's portion of the surgery (a two-day hospital stay and Laparoscopic Omentectomy) because "your plan does not cover this type of treatment." "Well that just sucks" were my thoughts exactly. December 13, 2022 came and we proceeded with the surgery. I had lost the battle prior to surgery, but I would continue the war that followed.

As I lay in the hospital less than 48 hours after waking up from SIXTEEN HOURS of anesthesia, I received a message from my friend keeping an eye on the mail for me at home. I had asked her to check if anything from insurance had come while I was away. Sure enough, on December 15th a letter came denying **all** of Dr. Aliu's portion by stating, "Purpose: This treatment is not approvable under the plan clinical criteria because there is no proof or not enough proof it improves health. For this reason, this request is denied as investigation. The associated hospital admission is considered not medically necessary. … The request tells us your doctor ordered a procedure to remove fat from under your skin (liposuction) to treat your left leg swelling (lymphedema)." Health insurance see the word "liposuction" and automatically jump to the conclusion of someone being overweight when that is very much not the case. At just 110 pounds, I was suffering from two liters of excess fluid in my left leg and foot, which affected the skin, overwhelmed the cells, and debilitated my muscles. Leaked lymph fluid was being targeted and removed for this procedure. Not fat. I sent another appeal, including a handwritten letter, medical papers, and conclusions about this surgery that had been tried and proven for the last 30 years. At this point we had a joke in the family that they all saw my name while sitting safely behind their desks and set my things aside with their big red stamp "denied" all over my cases. Obviously, my strong outcry pleading my case did not amuse them.

I sought solace in social media regarding the challenge I was facing. Not for attention, but for awareness. Awareness on how we, as a nation, are being treated and denied critical care from health insurance companies. It was overwhelming how much support I received to keep on fighting. My father could not be in Pennsylvania to help Team A and Team B with the immediate physical recovery, but he sure could help with insurance at home. After some research done by my father, I sent an external review request form to the State Corporation Commission Bureau of Insurance on December 27, 2022. This was likely going to be my last chance or else be in five-figures medical debt in my 20's. Then, we waited.

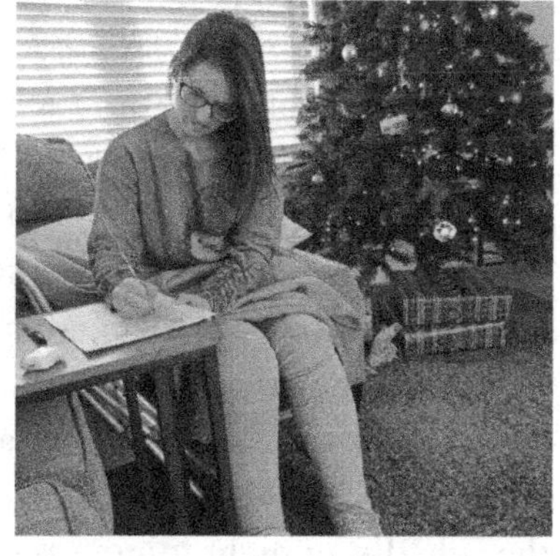

The day came on February 24, 2023. Three months of fighting, being denied by insurance seven times, going under the knife without coverage, and an appeal to the hierarchy of the State's insurances (an Independent Review Organization (IRO)). I received the final letter from my insurance stating: **"they have completed their review and approved coverage for the services. We will adjust all claims and/or authorizations with their decision."**

This was the most thrilling day of my life. **I WON!** The Independent Review Organization notes that the language of my procedure was reconstructive, not cosmetic as my private insurance was claiming. They also noted that "lipectomy or liposuction for the treatment of lymphedema…or lipedema is considered medically necessary when all of the following criteria are met…" In my case, I had met all criteria listed one through four as stated earlier.

Thinking back, this process may have seemed quick and not as lengthy as expected, but I want to emphasize the diligence and upkeep it took to have all the ducks in a row. Sending the necessary information to the IRO meant digging up everything. I sent them a binder worth of stuff. Go big or go home, right? I like to follow the rule of thumb that it is better to have too much information rather than not enough. That way they can decide what is not important and set it to the side. I sent eight to nine years' worth of receipts for custom-made compression garments, bandages, my pump, all my Occupational Therapy visits, and all my surgeries with Dr. Aliu. I sent them information and letters regarding my daily activity level and routine for taking care of my lymphoedema. I sent them everything they needed to know to make this decision.

The only unfortunate part of this was they approved the surgery itself, but the two to three day in-hospital stay was still denied. Long story short, the hospital continued to appeal for me and on April 1, 2024, I received a letter from my insurance company stating the inpatient services had finally been approved. When I received my first denial in November 2022, I did not imagine it would have led to an eighteen-month fight to approve the medical treatment I deserved. One thing is for sure, I was right to have my surgery on December 13,

2022. I don't regret one-bit not cancelling it and waiting. Life gets you nowhere when you sit back and wait. I became proactive and got the help I believed I desperately needed and deserved. My surgeon was in this fight with me every step of the way. He spent sixteen hours giving me back a life he believed I had earned and deserved. Saying "thank you" will never be enough. However, what I can do to thank him is to take care of myself and live my life to the fullest. And that I certainly do.

The Unbroken Gait

I will never forget the day in January 2020 when I received the text message "Soooo....do you still want your boy?" I was substitute teaching at the time because it allowed me to easily be away whenever I wanted to work at the racetrack during the summer or the race sales in the fall and winter. I was at my old high school in a math class. It was the last period of the day and there was absolutely no service in the building. It was the teacher's planning period, so I had no students, but I was sticking around to see my friend who was teaching health and PE down the hall. I was overjoyed and frantically texting back "YES!" at the speed of light. The text message wouldn't send. So, here I was running around the room high and low trying to send this message. I immediately texted Trey, at this time we had been together for three years, asking for forgiveness rather than permission. Yet, the first text still wouldn't go through. After the last bell I went power walking to my friend's office, trying to squeeze by a mob of high schoolers in this narrow hallway. Excited to say it out loud to someone. I yelled, "Kara, I have a horse!" She thought I was kidding. I had to repeat it for her to believe it. Having someone to run to right away made the excitement all too real. Trey was okay with this but wasn't quite as excited as everyone else was who would not have any responsibility for this lifelong commitment. (He loves our horse, but he won't show it).

Noble Descendant is such a light and joy in my life. He is such a gentle, caring and "in your pocket" kind of horse. I really got lucky with this one. I first met him in December of 2017 when he arrived at the farm. I already had experienced the reality of racehorses coming and going based on their training needs during the internship in Kentucky. So, I had told myself when I started the job, "Do not fall in love!" Well, sure enough when this little yearling colt walked off that trailer, I couldn't help but have an immediate likeness towards him. This was the beginning of developing a bond with the colt who eventually came into my ownership after his racing career. As I'm writing this book, he is now nine years old and I absolutely love that I have, almost literally, known him his whole life.

In the beginning I was a little worried about the physical commitment of owning a horse. I was also going through my surgeries which created periods of separation from him, but I knew that wouldn't last forever. In the end, every moment with him, whether it was a good leg day or a bad leg day, has been well worth it. He is more than just a hobby and more than something to ride and show. Having lymphoedema, he provides me a purpose. He teaches me lessons and he provides emotional support and sympathy. He teaches patience, trust, overcoming fears, confidence, listening skills, and boundaries. He also, most of all, keeps me on my toes.

I lost a lot of confidence one day when I was riding him in a grass field. This incident happened the second summer of having him. I *never* ride alone. That is my number one rule. So, on a nice day, I rode him in the flat grassy field that was next to the barn while the barn manager was cleaning stalls. She could easily keep an eye out. I stayed in a quadrant of the field working on circles and transitions. I was twenty-five minutes into the ride and happy with how Noble had behaved and focused, so I decided to call it a day. I thought, "He did so well let's reward him with a cool down lap around the field." I left my little quadrant area to take a lap around. Boom! Just like that, he shot off without warning like a bolt of lightning. Having no control of slowing down this Thoroughbred running full speed ahead I took a deep breath and told myself, "Just hold on." It having been quite a few years since I executed an emergency stop on a horse it came to mind to make a big circle. He couldn't go faster in a circle. Right? Well, that's when my mistake happened with unfortunate timing and not planning ahead. I started circling him, which was going fine, but I accidently steered him right into the one muddy patch of the field and it took a turn for the worst. Noble's feet slipped from under him crashing down to the ground. It happened so quickly I couldn't recollect the moment we were actually going down. One second I was turning him and the next I'm on the ground unable to breathe. My very first fear was him getting up and running loose with the reins and tack flying everywhere. I've seen a horse get tangled in the reins after losing their rider, so it has always been a fear in the back of my mind if I were to fall. However, he popped up fine, my feet slipped right out the stirrups, and I remember him taking a look back in the direction of the gate and then faced towards me and bent his head down to me on the ground. I rolled back over in too much pain to move and within seconds the barn manager was at my side.

Both Noble and I were completely okay after this accident. I was extremely sore for a few days but didn't have any concerns that I'd severely hurt anything. Unfortunately, I lost a lot of confidence after this ride. But I was very glad of how he acted just standing there as if saying, "I'm sorry Mom," instead of running off loose. The comical part of this story is after the fact when I was up and walking again, the manager said, "I saw you cantering and it looked so good!" I should have told her my intentions of the ride beforehand and mentioned if she sees any cantering it means I'm in trouble. I learned my lesson though. Noble was very young and still very green and he got a little excited. It happens, and it has happened many times since where he has bolted, but thanks to that day I have been able to handle it better and hold him back with each occurrence there on.

Another occurrence happened a couple years later when Noble and I were boarding at a different facility. This barn had electric fencing. The fenced area I used was much more comfortable to ride in being about the size of a large arena used as a small paddock. This paddock had wooden fencing with a live wire going across the top to keep horses from reaching each other over the fence. I had been riding in this paddock for a year and a half and not once did it occur to me that it was probably a good idea to make sure the electricity running through that thin wire was turned off. It may have been naïve of me, but I sure did learn my lesson.

I was riding on a nice day out. It was a very normal day and the barn manager was doing some afternoon chores so that I wasn't out there alone. I gave Noble a walk break halfway through our ride. We were walking along the fence and I was just taking the moment in. We had been working on suppleness and flexibility. A horse's head should be slightly bent to the inside. Well, we were still very much working on this. I saw him stick his nose out a little to the outside and it is one hundred percent my fault I did not correct him right away. And then there it was, the "pop" the live wire made at the touch of his nose. I've never experienced a one-eighty so quickly in my life. I heard that zap and thought to myself, "Oh shit!" I was facing one direction and without warning I was in the other direction then I was looking up at the sky. I hit the ground so hard flat on my back. Thankfully, my bottom took the brunt of the fall where I have all the cushion. In a matter of seconds my barn manager was hunched over me feeling terrible that the fence was plugged in. I was the one riding, so I told her not to feel bad for it was my responsibility. I just didn't think of it, but I guarantee you I did every time after that! We both lifted our heads and Noble was running like a mad man. He would stop, stare at us, then run off again. Stop, stare at us, run off again. I asked, "I already know the answer to this, but do I have to get back on?" Obviously, the answer was yes. Poor Noble shocking himself resulted in taking a solid five minutes to catch him. He was fine though. It just took him by surprise. After I got myself up and seeing straight again, I first lunged him, settled him down and ended our ride with a nice walk under saddle. All was well with the world.

The message I want to get across through this chapter is not to be scared of horses, animals or anything of the like at all. The importance of this story is to live your life to the fullest. Enjoy the things you love and don't let your lymphoedema, disease, illness or fears keep you from living life to the utmost fullest. Thanks to my surgeon and occupational therapist I am living my best life. My surgeon encourages me to live the life that makes me happy. If I were to get hurt in any kind of capacity, then we would figure it out. After all the hard work he has done to reconstruct my lymphatic system, he supports and encourages me to go after my dreams.

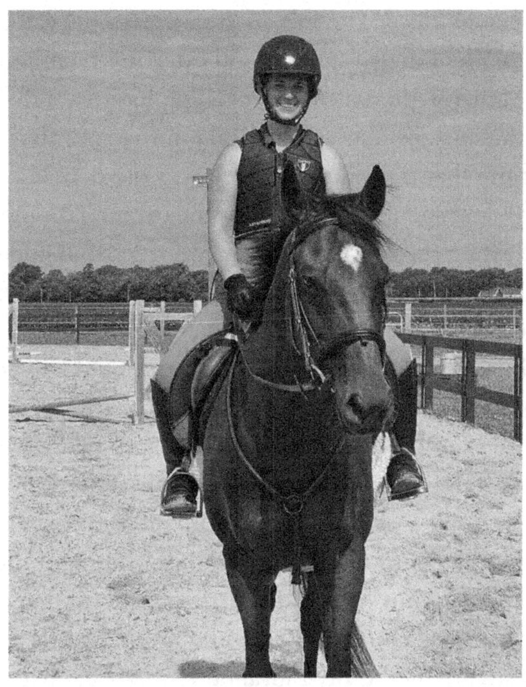

How important is physical activity for lymphoedema? Well, according to Macmillan Cancer Support, moving your body "Works your muscles, which increases the flow of lymph fluid through the lymphatic system and helps move it away from the swollen area."[1] If you do not have lymphoedema, according to the Centers for Disease Control and Prevention, physical activity is still important because it can "improve your brain health, help manage weight, reduce the risk of disease, strengthen bones and muscles, and improve your ability to do

---

1 Macmillan Cancer Support. 2025. *Managing lymphoedema with physical activity. https://www.macmillan.org.uk/cancer-information-and-support/impacts-of-cancer/lymphoedema/managing-lymphoedema-with-exercise#:~:text=Physical%20activity%3A,improving%20your%20range%20of%20movement.*

every day activities."[2] Having my horse gives me a purpose to stay moving and active not just to better my health and keep me sane, but for the better of my lymphatic system as well. Moving the muscles acts as a natural pump to pump the fluid. I would argue that it is more beneficial for me than going home from work and spending the rest of the evening on the couch.

So, despite the scary moments and rides that end up with me face planting in the ground, being a rider provides movement and exercise which I need to manage the lymphoedema. Having him also teaches me to be goal oriented and celebrate success no matter how small. Having Noble Descendant gives me a cause I am passionate about not just to take care of myself, but to take care of him as well. The activity doesn't always have to be a riding lesson. We could go on a relaxing trail ride or give him a bath and hand graze him in the sun or even just groom him. We could work on ground manners and different cues or I could just walk him around while talking to him. Horses are incredibly therapeutic and great listeners. So, think to yourself, what is your "why" that keeps you going?

All these things paired with my surgeries have made physical activity so much easier and less painful than my pre-surgeries lifetime. Pre-surgeries I was at the barn only a couple times a week with no motivation and trying to manage pain. Grooming was a burden and riding was near impossible. Post-surgeries I have gone to the barn nearly every day. My physical motivation isn't the only thing improved but my mental and emotional health has improved as well. Grooming is easier and riding is fun! That's the way life should be, right?

---

[2] U.S. Centers for Disease Control and Preventiom. 2024. *Benefits of Physical Activity.* 24 April. *https://www.cdc.gov/physical-activity-basics/benefits/?CDC_AAref_Val=https://www.cdc.gov/physicalactivity/basics/pa-health/index.htm.*

This brings me to a good point that animals are the best listeners. They are a blank canvas who have no judgement. They provide their own secret language to tell you all the answers you need to know. Or, they provide a simple listening ear if you're not looking for any answers. Or possibly the look of, "Excuse me, but it's dinner time" is always plausible too. My husband and I got his first puppy in the fall of 2023. A spirited chocolate American Labrador. This was my husband's first duck dog, so yes, we did consider him his dog. Our new lab puppy, Waylon, has been another emotional support to have at home as much as Noble has been. My favourite part is ganging up on my husband with two pairs of puppy dog eyes beating down on him for whatever we want. I mean, how can you resist that? An adorable lab face and the adorable wife? Impossible I say. We may have lost, or sacrificed, a few pairs of socks, a ruined hat, teeth marks in almost everything, but coming home from work every day with his cute, long limbs hanging over the couch and that little otter tail wagging makes all the messes well worth it.

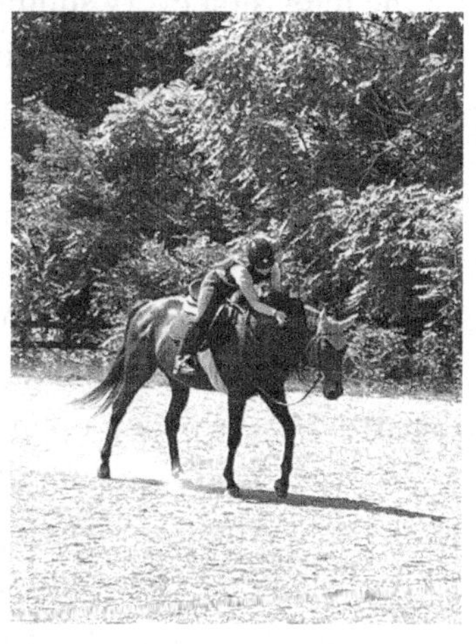

Over the years, I have thought a lot about what kind of equestrian I could have been, or be, without the lymphoedema. As an equestrian with two healthy legs, I know I would do great things with horses and my riding. However, I became a good rider and a good horsewoman in a short period of time. I did this through silent pain. What I thought back then was the edema was holding me back. What I know now is there was a bigger plan lying ahead.

You may be wondering how I got into the Thoroughbred industry in the first place. That alone is a very interesting story that I am so proud of. In the horse racing industry, it is very common to be born and raised in this field. Not only was I not born nor raised in it, but I was raised in the city and nowhere near horses. I always loved horses and the thought of riding, but my parents had no idea what to do or where to go. So, I never did the horse camp thing and I never did the 4-H club. I just always loved the idea of horses and watched the big races on the television every summer. I had no idea the meaning of the horses and their contribution to the industry and agriculture. I just loved the idea of going fast.

My senior year of high school, I was recruited to play softball in college. While on a private tour with the coaches over winter break, we were talking about the programmes and demanding schedule. A comment came up regarding their specialty programmes, being the equestrian and aviation departments. Growing up in the city and never around horses, I never thought in a million years you could get a degree in horses. I attended this same university and graduated four and a half years later with a major in history and minor in equestrian studies. As a minor, I was not required to take an internship to graduate. However, I wanted to. By my senior year of college I thought to myself, "I did it. I found my way to horses and have established a foundation in horsemanship." But we only did dressage and hunters/jumpers. As a career, I wanted to be in Thoroughbred horse racing. This is what led me to go to Kentucky spring break of 2016 to find an internship. Sure enough, I landed an incredible opportunity at a highly successful farm and award-winning enterprise. Little introvert me, with lymphoedema in my right leg, took control of my future and went off to find opportunity instead of sitting at home waiting for opportunity to find me.

During the time in Kentucky, I got to know family on my dad's side whom I never really knew before. I am very grateful to have developed a special relationship in my adulthood with these family members in a very special place in Kentucky.

Fast forward to fall of 2017. A friend at the time shared a job posting with me for a Thoroughbred training facility in the neighboring county. A few short weeks later, after Thanksgiving, I began work for this trainer as a groom. Little did I know at the time I was making new lifelong racing friends. This is also where I met Noble when he came out of the trailer for training two weeks later. I wanted to work there forever. I wanted that to be it and be my "forever job" because I loved it so much. After a while my boss could see I truly had a passion for this industry. I wasn't just a horse-loving local wanting a job on a farm. I learned quickly this industry is all about networking. I gradually became more extraverted and was no longer the shy little Kiersten I used to be. However, my lymphoedema increasingly got worse. The trainer got me started working the horse sales in Maryland. The consignment I worked for is another connection I have grown close to. I seemed to do well, and my size was perfect for showing the young horses. While talking at the sales, I wanted to learn and grow in experience, so I connected with another consignment in Kentucky. So, for the next couple years I bounced around to working at the farm, sales in Maryland, the winter sales in Kentucky, and at my home state's racetrack during the summer once it reopened in 2019. At the time, I thought I was living the dream. In my mid-twenties I was having so much fun! But my lymphoedema was getting worse and I had to come to terms.

I had a hard time figuring it out. I worked SO HARD to get into the racing industry from the outside. But I didn't know what kind of careers were out there and what was out there that would work for the swelling. Everything I wanted to be I couldn't do because of this disease. I landed a full-time job at the racetrack in 2021 in the finance department. I was thrilled at the time because I was working at a racetrack. I thought I had made it, but two years later and reality hit. I was working at the track, but the work had no effect on the horses. After three years at the track, I found my current job. And day one I knew this was it. This was the job, the career for me, and I am able to effectively manage my swelling while doing it.

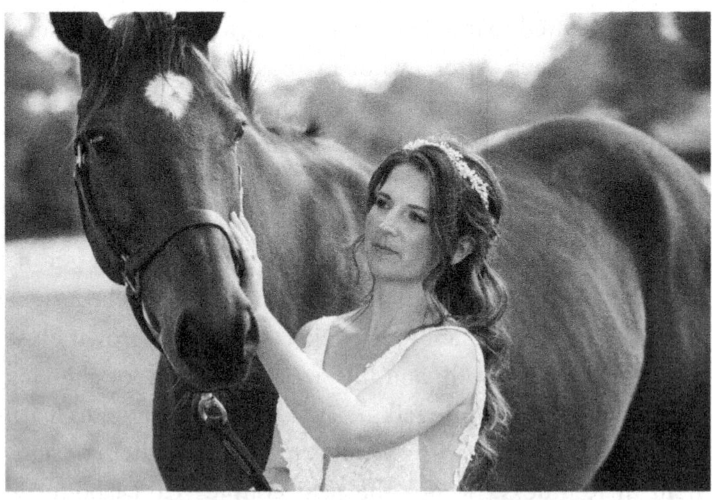

Ashley Nicole Photography

Travelling

Living with lymphoedema has made travelling a huge challenge. How many of us have found ourselves on the road or in a hotel room when we realised we forgot to pack a necessary item? It could be a toothbrush, some socks, or even clothes for the right weather. No big deal, anything of the like can be bought at the nearest convenience store, boutique, Target, or Walmart. For us Lymphies though it's not that simple. Am I guilty of travelling and forgetting compression garments, a stockinette or a wrap for bandaging? Yes, yes, and definitely yes in my less organised days. It's more than devastating. It's detrimental to our care. Our vacation just went from exciting to possibly miserable. We can't get these things at any local store. Maybe one can be lucky and find a specialty pharmacy who sell circular knit stockings off the shelf. However, for the most part, all of our items for our care are special ordered. It's not fun forgetting anything when you leave the house for a trip of any kind.

This leads me to bring up how I prepare to travel for my lymphoedema. Several years ago, my parents gifted me the best Christmas present a young adult could not know to ask for: a luggage set. This was completely not on my radar and I didn't know at the time how nice it would be to have decent luggage bags stowed away instead of my little kid hot pink bag. I was so surprised and loved it. They got me a four-piece set that came with the big suitcase, medium suitcase, a carry-on, and a small bag. It all matched and was part of the same set from Macy's. When I saw the carry-on and the nifty pockets and compartments it had my very first thought was, "This is perfect for my leg stuff." I immediately found a home in the bag for extras of anything I could possibly need on the road; a couple stockinettes, an old toe cap, toe wraps, gloves, lotion, measuring tape, and more! The bag was also carry-on size for airplanes and works perfectly for traveling by plane. Your all-important leg stuff can't get lost if it stays with you at your seat! This technique for traveling, by car or plane, has been a life saver. Strategically packed, it fits two sets of bandages and my flat knit compression garments for both legs. This is something I would highly recommend for any Lymphie! It takes a lot of stress away and keeps Lymphie stuff packed in one place. Plus, as mentioned before, you can keep extras of the little things in case anything is forgotten packing in a hurry.

In recent history, 2022 post-surgery to present, I have found it much more bearable to travel by car sitting in the back seat with my legs elevated by pillows. Regardless of the length of drive, whether it be one hour or twelve hours, it has significantly aided in reducing swelling from travel. I can also last much longer without needing a break to stretch my legs. This helps out the hubby because he is not a fan of making stops. This has helped with our trips because instead of stopping every hour for a break from being cramped in the front seat we can now go a couple hours or longer with me comfortably stretched out in the back seat before I need a walking break. Considering how much time we spend on the road, whether to see my surgeon, enjoy our hobbies, or to see family, I truly believe this tip has aided in my surgeries being such a success.

I also travel exclusively wrapped in bandages. If I'm in the car longer than an hour in my flat knit garments my legs get very angry. I can feel them swelling up and the skin getting tight. It's quite miserable, but one of those things that come with lymphoedema that you just have to deal with. It is a full-time job—twenty-four hours a day, seven days a week, three hundred and sixty-five days a year. If I am traveling by car for more than a couple hours, I plan my day to travel in bandages.

Taking a Stand

There are so many things in this world that need to change. Everyone has their passion and opinion on what is most important. My passion and priority is, obviously, lymphoedema. So many things need to change, but one quarter into the twenty-first century and we are finally on the right path.

As of January 1, 2024, the Lymphedema Treatment Act (LTA) went into effect in the United States. In short, this law provides the necessary coverage for medically necessary compression supplies for patients under Medicare. This is a *huge* step in the right direction thanks to the founding of the Lymphedema Advocacy Group.[3] It took this group fourteen years to get this bill passed.

This brings me to what still needs to change. (All based off my opinion of course). More health insurance companies and plans need to adopt this coverage. My first argument is that insurances, as I have been told, do not have a code for the toe cap connected to thigh high flat-knit compression garments. This means, when I order this garment, even though it is physically one piece, it is counted as two pieces. When

3 *https://lymphedemaadvocacygroup.org/*

I am docked for two pieces that is two units of the eight that my insurance plan will cover. So, to sum it up, when I order two sets of garments—four physical items—insurance docks me for eight items. The insurance policy is an arbitrary limitation that directly impacts my care and makes it difficult to manage my condition. The system is cruel, but what can we do to modify this?

My second argument is the quantity of units per limb. In my experiences this past decade, no matter what insurance or plan I had, I have been limited to coverage of eight units total. This was not a problem when I had unilateral lymphoedema. However, this did become a problem when I developed bilateral lymphoedema. When I needed eight units for one limb, I now need for two limbs. How can I take care of myself and stay out of the hospital and live a quality life with such restrictions on my level of care? I know other patients who have lymphoedema in more than two limbs. How do they do it? I ask myself this all the time. How have we, as a society, have gone so long accepting this lack of care from our country? This is all my completely biased opinion, of course.

My mom once said to me, "it takes you over an hour to get ready?" There was a time in my life I could wake up and be ready within ten minutes. I remember in my travel softball days I could be out the door in less than ten minutes. Unfortunately, those days are *long* gone. With lymphoedema it takes me ten minutes alone just to get garments on! I have extra steps to take to get ready for the day: stretching, MLD, and compression. I am also not a springy teenager any longer, so I do not like to rush. If there is time to roll my bandages before leaving the house, I like to take advantage of doing so. This way I have that much more time for myself in the evening. It makes my evening a bit easier for after-work activities.

So yes, yes it does take me over an hour to get ready for my day.

I want to change the game for lymphoedema. Even if it only affects a fraction of the world. To a single person, it could be their whole world.

The Weight I Accepted

Acceptance, "approval." (Dictionary.com).

I don't know how to explain it, but it's hard work being miserable. The disease brought out hatred, crushed my spirit, and changed my views on quality of life and the world. It broke my character and shattered my soul. But, one day, I became miserable being miserable. I realised something needed to change and I didn't want to be that person with a dark cloud over their head anymore. For years I put myself in a deep, dark hole with no intentions of ever coming out. I was angry, upset, confused, and discouraged. I finally said, "enough is enough" to the bad attitude and my unhappy lifestyle. I had the support, but at the end of the day it was me that had to take care of myself. Mentally and emotionally, I was stuck in a deep, dark well rising with water. There were hands from family, friends, even strangers, reaching down trying to help; however, they could not reach me without me equally wanting to get out of the well. I had two choices: I could either allow the lymphoedema to slowly drown me over time or I could reach up and find a way to grab the hands of those wanting to pull me out. After several years of drowning, I finally chose to reach up for the heavens and get pulled out of the well. I became my own saving grace and my life has been so much better ever since.

Acceptance of this disease was very difficult to overcome. As you have read, it was not an overnight transition. However, the first step had to be an overnight realization: looking in the mirror and telling myself something had to change. I live with my disease, I conquered my disease, I overcame my disease. I had to accept the loss of normal and create a new normal. My lymphoedema may force some of the decisions I make, but it does not define the person I am going to be. Acceptance never means accepting defeat. It's accepting reality. It is accepting that sometimes you may need a little bit of help. And asking for help is not a sign of weakness. I believe it is a sign of strength when you are aware of your weaknesses. We all have areas we need help in and there is absolutely nothing wrong with that. Coming to this realization, I'm not fighting with my body anymore—I'm working with it. Like a relationship between a man and wife, a clown fish and an anemone, sharks and remora, or coyote and badger. It requires give and take from each party. Some days the lymphoedema requires more and my own needs less. Other days I require more and my lymphoedema has to receive less. I listen to my body to make those decisions. Acceptance has taught me to put my health first. No amount of money is worth my mental health. No opportunity is worth my physical health. And no person is worth my emotional health. One can't take care of others if one can't take care of themselves. It doesn't do anyone any good to push themselves beyond repair and into a hospital bed or even six-feet under. Ask for help! See the doctor. Ask questions. Put yourself first. Facing reality has taught me this invaluable lesson.

Change is scary, but you don't have to change. Lymphoedema doesn't have to change who you are as a person or what you enjoy in life. Instead of changing your lifestyle, transform it. Transform your routine. Transform your interests. Transform your activities. By accepting this disease, you are capable of altering the way you go about it instead of changing who you are.

Lymphoedema has brought people in my life whom I would have never met without it. It gave me a job opportunity I would have never aspired to do. It taught me to enjoy what I have because I may not have it the same way or even at all one day. It has also taught me patience, organizational skills, and how to fight for something that I believe in.

There was a day on Instagram in 2024 when a certified lymphoedema therapist messaged me asking, "Since your diagnosis in 2014, what's been most helpful for you in managing it? Or are there any areas where you're still looking for support?" After a decade of lymphoedema life my immediate thoughts were, "Honestly, what has been the most helpful in managing my lymphoedema is acceptance. Acceptance of the disease led me to start taking care of myself. Acceptance of changing the routine led me to figure out better ways to manage it. Accepting the inevitability of bad days has significantly helped me ease my mental self-criticism. I became kinder to myself. I know that's probably not what most people would expect as an answer, but for me, accepting the cards I was given has opened up so many wonderful things in my life." The tools you have in order to manage the chronic swelling are only so useful if you don't accept why you need to use these tools.

I have built a life that feels like summer camp every day. Chores don't feel like chores anymore. Running errands aren't a burden anymore. I am so happy and so joyful. I have the energy level of a 16-year-old again. I have been able to accomplish all this because of scientific advancement, my surgeon, my occupational therapist, my medical team, my support system, my attitude, and my dedication to *myself.* All my life I was never one to make New Year's resolutions or to set goals. However, in 2023 I set a huge goal for myself—to not overdo it. To not overwork myself. My goal was to become a better listener. Listen to instructions, listen to my body, listen to nature and all things that surrounded me. By August 2023 my life had been so much fun; so much better. Life is joyful and exciting now. I opened up a whole new world for my quality of living. To my mental, physical, and emotional well-being I have to give so much credit to my surgeon, Dr. Oluseyi Aliu. He was someone that knew how to help me and how to educate me. With the surgeries, he laid a foundation for my life to improve. He essentially handed me the baton to be happier living with this disease and by God I took that baton and I ran. I am still running. He spent 16 hours in the operating room, which was not planned, to make my life better. He chose to make the rest of his week more difficult in order to make the rest of my life immeasurably better. He provided me with a new attitude on life and on outcomes. With this new attitude I turned my disease into my destiny.

Coincidentally enough at the very end of 2023, I came across the most beautiful movie on Netflix called *All the Light We Cannot See.* It was about a young girl named Marie who was blind and alone during WWII in a German occupied small French town. Despite the blindness, she was surviving on her own in a three-story house and even going as far as walking through the city for food with no assistance but her memory and hearing. She listened for every voice in the air, creak from the floor, and whisper through the walls. It was amazing how she embodied "everything has a voice" (as she stated in a scene). As I learned to listen to my body in 2023, to really listen, I learned that everything has a voice. I have a voice. **We** have a voice. As a community, I do find it important to come together and use our voice. Whether that be reaching out asking for a shoulder to cry on during the bad days, to fight the insurance claim that was denied for our lymphoedema needs, or reaching out to your local legislator on why it is so important to change laws to provide care for our needs. We need to speak and to speak loudly. Just like the Whos of Whoville in Dr. Seuss' *Horton Hears a Who*, Horton advocates for the tiny town on the red clover to prevent their destruction by the antagonists of the story. They all scream to the heavens to create noise and together they made a difference. Lymphoedema may have taken a few things away from me, but it cannot, and will not, take away my voice. We speak out. We let others know they can thrive. We let others know they can survive. We let others know it is possible to conquer the lymphoedema. We let others know they are not alone.

Every day we have a choice to make. We can make the good choice or the bad one. We can make the right decision or the wrong. We can make positive decisions or negative ones. I used to choose the negativity, hatred, and depression. Now I choose to live. To survive. To thrive. I choose to take care of myself. I choose to embrace imperfection in the face of adversity. I choose to see every detail within the bigger picture. I became my own saving grace choosing to make a difference for my health and my attitude. I may not be a celebrity, or an influencer, or rich, or famous. I don't claim to be anyone of social importance, but I'm not a no one. I am a someone. I am someone to my husband, my parents, and my brother. I am a someone to my nieces, my in-laws, and friends. I am a someone to my doctors, my surgeon, and my occupational therapist. But most important of all, **I am a someone for myself**.

Life is for the living, and it takes happiness to feel alive. So, surmount the obstacle put upon you and pursue the life your soul is meant to thrive. After many years of wandering, I finally found my Promised Land, and it is beautiful. I call my Promised Land "Acceptance."

I have lymphoedema and I have made it my mission to discover the legacy I will leave behind.

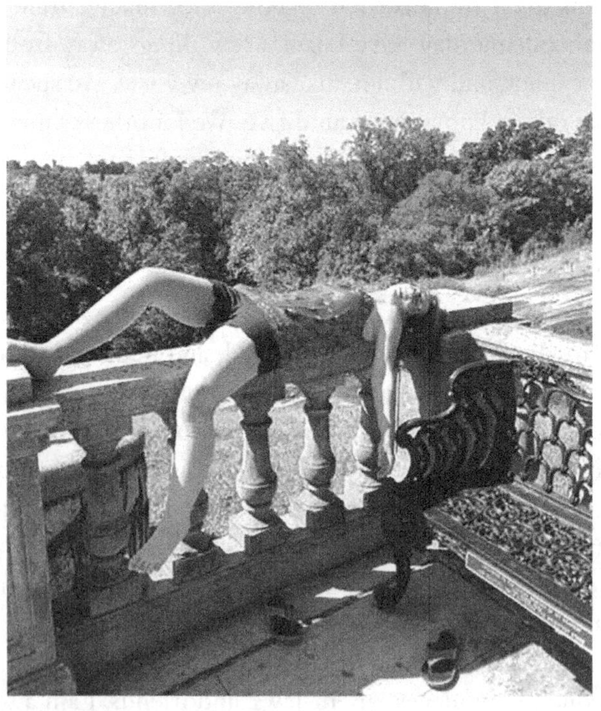

"If you would not be forgotten, as soon as you were dead and rotten, either write things worth reading, or do things worth writing."

–BENJAMIN FRANKLIN:
POOR RICHARD'S ALMANAC

ACKNOWLEDGEMENTS

Betty with the Lymphedema Podcast —
www.thelymphedemapodcast.com

Sydney Gay — Editor

Trey Wall III — Husband of author

Michele Estes —Mother of author

Michael Estes — Father of author

Matthew & Erika Estes — Brother & Sister-in-Law of author

Dr. Aliu, MD — Plastic and Reconstructive Surgeon

CLT Bell — Occupational Therapist, CLT

FNP JK — Family Nurse Practitioner

Dr. M — Physician

All my Lymphoedema friends

Photos

Ashley Nicole Photography
Dr. Aliu, MD
Family & Friends

ABOUT THE AUTHOR

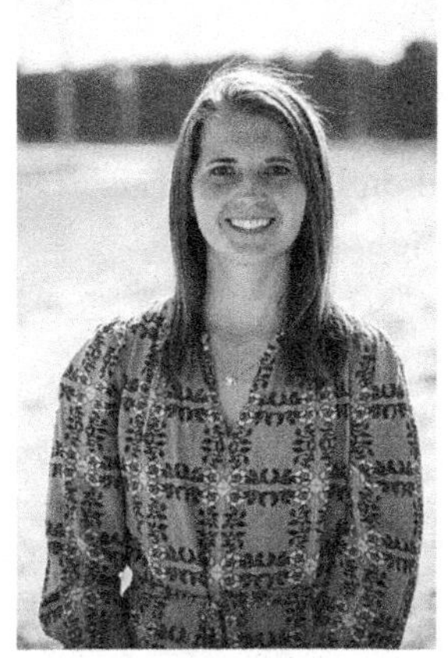

Ashley Nicole Photography

Kiersten Wall is the author of *The Weight We Carry: Navigating Life with Lympoedema.* She has a passion for Thoroughbred horse racing and spreading lymphoedema awareness. In the late 90's Kiersten's family moved to England which opened up a unique appreciation to culture, history, and opportunity. You will find subtle hints of her early education throughout her writing. Growing up, Kiersten bounced around with different dreams not knowing what she wanted to do. Whether it was a professional baseball player, jockey, a paleontologist, photographer, or a graphic designer, horses were always a constant deep down in her heart.

Her lymphoedema journey became intertwined with finding her niche in the Thoroughbred industry. After giving it a try as a groom, brief opportunity as a rider, horse sales showman, and payroll at a racetrack, she landed herself the best gig of all—promoting and supporting the Virginia Thoroughbred horse in her home state. The drive she has for the horses, association's members, the horsemen, and the industry is immeasurable. The passion gets her through all the good days and the bad with lymphoedema.

Other activities Kiersten enjoys in her spare time are preparing and competing in horse shows with her Off Track Thoroughbred (OTTB), spending time with her dogs, and enjoying every moment of life with her husband. When they have some free time between race seasons and events, Kiersten and her husband sneak away to experience new adventures.

Kiersten's journey can be followed on her Instagram @8furlongs_of_lymph.

Made in United States
Orlando, FL
14 April 2026